Ethics
in
MIDWIFERY

Shirley R. Jones

SRN, SCM, ADM, Cert.Ed.(FE),
Teaching (Midwifery), MA

Midwifery Tutor
Birmingham and Solihull College of Nursing and Midwifery, and
Tutor–Counsellor, Distance Learning Centre
South Bank University
London

M Mosby

Copyright © 1994 Mosby–Year Book Europe Ltd
Reprinted 1995 by Mosby, an imprint of Times Mirror International Publishers Ltd
Printed and bound in Great Britain by Biddles Ltd, Guildford and King's Lynn
ISBN 0 7234 1971 X

A CIP catalogue record for this book is available from the British Library.

For full details of all Times Mirror International Publishers Ltd titles please write to
Times Mirror International Publishers Ltd, Lynton House, 7–12 Tavistock Square, London
WC1H 9LB, England.

For my Dad

Tom Phillips

who was very excited about the completion
of this book but who sadly died before its
publication

T04083   1742
         J

CONTENTS

ACKNOWLEDGEMENTS

I would like to offer my sincere thanks to the following people, without whom I could not have achieved my dissertation, which was the forerunner to this book:

To my husband Alan, not only for his support and encouragement, but also for his practical advice and assistance in producing the final document.

To my mum Dilys, for the considerable amount of proof-reading and for her encouragement and domestic assistance.

To Bobbie (Calliope Farsides), for her immense support and advice.

To the Birmingham and Solihull College of Midwifery Education and Training, for supporting me in my studies.

Last but not least come my children, Darren and Kerri, for sharing their mum with books and a computer and making numerous cups of coffee.

PART ONE

ETHICAL THEORY

INTRODUCTION

(Note: Midwives, in this text, should be considered to be male or female; generally, feminine pronouns have been used only for ease of writing. The midwife in Chapter 6 is a man.)

Midwifery students will be embarking on an adult education course, perhaps for the first time, and as adult learners must be responsible for their own learning. They should be self-directed, taking an active part in seeking, through their own and their peers' efforts, to broaden their knowledge; they should receive tutorial assistance that is tailored more to their individual needs. The students will come to the course with a wide variety of backgrounds and experiences—in the case of post-registration students there will be some similarities in professional experience, whereas the pre-registration students will possibly be very different. These differences can be used to broaden the outlook of the group as a whole and to give different perspectives on various issues, if they are given the chance to discuss freely.

When in the clinical areas, the students will have to learn to identify the ethical issues, consider the possible actions that could be taken, then select the appropriate course. In the interests of safety, as these situations often need decisions to be made quickly, it would be more acceptable for the public—and less threatening for the students—to simulate situations in the classroom. This could be done by role play but it does not necessarily require practical simulation; the author's choice would be to use carefully constructed case studies. These can then be used individually or in small groups, with feedback to a larger group if appropriate, or main group discussion if numbers are not prohibitive.

If the ethics module of the reader's course is to be assessed, then written work could be practised around the cases, perhaps using the questions as a basis for formulating an answer plan. This may encourage additional reading including the consideration of newspaper articles, women's magazines and television programmes, not only 'known texts'. This may well indicate the tendency for one-sided views to be reported by the media.

Where to include ethics in the education programme is debatable. It could be argued that it is a basic need of the students and that, as such, it should feature as a large component at the beginning of training. It would be correct to say this of anatomy, physiology or even psychology—they are equally important for different reasons. However, the author considers it more worthwhile to thread ethics through the whole course, starting with the basic principles of everyday practice—such as accountability and confidentiality—working through to more sophisticated principles at appropriate stages of training. Some aspects could be studied as individual topics, which would then be applied to relevant situations. This is just one view, however, and the intention of this book is that it should be used according to the desires of the individual who wishes to try it.

It is common practice among many tutors in midwifery (but by no means all) to start everything with a definition. The author will continue this practice by defining the title of this work: *Ethics in Midwifery*.

On first hearing the word 'ethics' many people feel they know what it means but would then have difficulty explaining it. Looking at a parallel profession, Gillon (1990) explains medical ethics, briefly, as:

... the critical study of moral problems arising in the context of medical practice.

Although the power bases in medicine and midwifery are different—and therefore cannot usually be substituted directly for each other—it would seem reasonable for our purposes to substitute midwifery for 'medical' in this definition. In doing this it is necessary to consider what is meant by 'moral problems'. These should be interpreted as problems involving moral values: the rights and wrongs, the 'oughts' and 'ought nots' of our practices. Perhaps a clearer explanation was given by Wilday when delivering the Eighth Dame Rosalind Paget Memorial Lecture 'Ethics in Midwifery' (1989). She explained it as being 'the study of the underlying reasons for deciding what is best in the face of conflicting choices'. The 'best', as used here, includes both prudential and moral considerations. It may be considered prudent, for instance, to inform a woman that she may require a caesarean section for a particular complication; moral considerations, however, would suggest that she be given sufficient information, and opportunity to question, in order to give or withhold informed consent.

Anyone who is not familiar with a midwife's sphere of practice may understandably question the need for ethics at all in the educational programme. Many people think that doctors make all the decisions and so midwives would rarely face conflicting choices, in fact midwifery is a parallel profession to obstetrics and its members may be concerned with the dilemmas presented by conflicts in a wide range of issues:

• Preconception care
• Genetic counselling
• Genetic engineering
• Infertility
• The reproductive revolution (including surrogacy, etc.)
• Screening for fetal abnormality
• Termination of pregnancy
• Contraception
• Advice and care throughout pregnancy, labour and the postnatal period
• Care of abnormal babies
• Care of preterm babies
• Care of 'damaged' or dying babies
• Care of handicapped mothers
• Care of dying mothers (including life-support)
• Care of very young mothers
• Incest
• Child abuse.

Nurses, midwives and health visitors are governed by the UK Central Council for Nursing, Midwifery and Health Visiting (UKCC) who have produced the *Code of Professional Conduct* (1992), among other leaflets, which guide their practice. Midwives, however, have two further documents to abide by: the *Midwives' Rules* (1991a) and the *Midwife's Code of Practice* (1991b). There is also a document produced by the Royal College of Midwives regarding ethics in midwifery practice: *Practical Guidance for Midwives Facing Ethical or Moral Dilemmas* (1989). Doctors also have a number of codes and declarations that guide their practice, and it is always possible that conflicts will arise precisely because each profession is practising what they think their code requires of them.

The intention in writing this book is to assist in the education of midwifery students, while not excluding other health care students. It may also be of use to others involved in the education and training of such students—such as clinical midwives and tutors. It is hoped that it will be particularly useful to those who feel threatened by the inclusion of ethics in the curriculum, if only to highlight examples and explain certain principles; however, it is not intended that this should be a definitive work.

The book is arranged in two parts: Part One consists of the ethical theory, giving the background to the possible reasons for certain ethical decision making. Part Two consists mainly of six case studies, in separate chapters, with relevant questions and the discussion points surrounding these questions.

In each chapter there is a 'Further discussion' section and suggested reading is listed, in addition to the references (with bibliographical entries) which some readers may choose to pursue. By using these case studies it is envisaged that readers will be able to apply the ethical theory from Part One. The case studies have been ordered according to the perceived needs of students; for instance, it is assumed that the principle of confidentiality will need to be addressed before the management of resources, therefore 'Confidentiality' appears first and 'Resource allocation' is last. Further information regarding the case studies can be found at the beginning of Part Two and a glossary of terms used has been included to aid clarification. The characters used in the case studies and illustrative examples are not intended to depict any particular race or social class, names having been selected at random. Readers will also find that the author has made use of some situations that are not purely midwifery ones. Some situations have an obstetric bias; no apology is made for this as, in practice, these are often the areas of most concern to students and qualified midwives. In fact this was a definite request from midwives canvassed by the author at the start of this work. There are also some situations that are 'non-health care' ones but which serve to highlight or clarify the principles, without creating a confusion of issues.

REFERENCES

Gillon, R. (1990) Teaching medical ethics: Impressions from the USA, in *Medicine, Medical Ethics and the Value of Life* (ed. P. Byrne), John Wiley and Sons, Chichester, p.90.

RCM (1989) *Practical Guidance for Midwives Facing Ethical or Moral Dilemmas*, London.

UKCC (1991a) *Handbook of Midwives' Rules.*

UKCC (1991b) *A Midwife's Code of Practice*, 3rd edn.

UKCC (1992) *Code of Professional Conduct for the Nurse, Midwife and Health Visitor*, 2nd edn.

Wilday, R.J. (1989) Ethics in midwifery. *Midwives' Chronicle*, 176.

ETHICAL THEORY

IS ETHICAL REASONING PART OF EVERYDAY LIFE?

It seems obvious that ethical reasoning is an essential component of life if we choose to live in society with other individuals. The completely amoral individual is a very rare specimen, therefore the great majority of people are capable of recognizing moral dilemmas and conflicts when they arise. They are recognized as a part of life, irrespective of a commitment to solving them or success in doing so. In most situations people act intuitively if their upbringing and general socialization has laid down 'good' principles. There are situations, however, when conscious practical decisions need to be made that are not intuitive, for example, when buying a bottle of shampoo people would prudently select one suitable for their own or their families' hair type(s) but morally they may consider buying a brand where animal testing has not been used. Likewise with buying petrol—for many people it is no longer just a matter of 'filling up with four star' as was once the case but of considering the effect of lead emissions polluting the air.

There are of course the more serious situations, such as the teenager with a drug-addicted friend (see pp.21), the relative or neighbour who suspects someone of child abuse, or the person who drinks and drives. It could be argued that at the time of driving while under the influence of alcohol, the driver is not completely rational (this surely is why it is inadvisable) and therefore is not actually choosing to commit this 'bad' action. Another consideration is that if motorists have driven to wherever they are drinking—without making adequate provision for the return journey—then the choice was made either when leaving home or when ordering or accepting the drinks that caused them to be over the limit.

WHAT IS ETHICS?

Ethics is the application of the processes and theories of moral philosophy to a 'real' situation. It is concerned with the basic principles and concepts that guide human beings in thought and action, and which underlie their values. This is certainly affected by the various agencies involved in a person's upbringing—such as family, friends, school and any religious beliefs. Adults not only draw on these set values, but encounter situations that prompt them to confirm, alter or deny them. This would generally not occur as a 'Sunday afternoon' activity, rather in an ongoing, almost subconscious, way.

As philosophy divides into various branches, so too does ethics; it would appear to have three accepted parts:

• *Meta-ethics (ethics)* This is moral philosophy conducted at the most abstract level and it concerns the nature and status of moral thought and the language used. What is meant by 'good', 'bad' or 'happiness', how do people *know* that one decision is better than another, are there any moral truths or are there only individuals' moral opinions? (Norman, 1988.) Are there such things as facts relating to morality?

• *Ethical/moral theory* This attempts to formulate a procedure or mechanism for solving ethical problems. Most of today's adults, as schoolchildren, learned formulae for solving mathematical problems; it could be suggested that the majority felt that they were of little use to them—purely a means of psychological torture that the mathematics teachers inflicted on them! It is probable that many people have used very few of these formulae since adolescence, unless working out areas for carpets and curtains, or percentages. The reason for this, surely, is the irrelevance of some of them in the everyday lives of most people; after all, how often do *you* need to find the area of a pyramid?

Ethical problems are obviously different. They remain with us throughout life in various forms, they require decisions to be made—sometimes urgently— that will have consequences other than a tick or cross in a mathematics book. It could, therefore, be seen as essential to find a formula which can be drawn on whenever such a situation arises. Some contemporary philosophers, however, reject the need for formal theories which can then be applied to every situation, or a list of principles that should always be referred to. They prefer to develop the moral sensibilities of individuals so that they can discern the rights and wrongs as they arise, and within the circumstances surrounding them. This viewpoint is called particularism.

• *Practical ethics* This deals with the specific, everyday issues that occur in life generally, and also in defined areas such as medicine and business. Everyday issues cannot be divorced from the more defined issues, however, as people do not shed their personal moral codes (for daily living and the interaction between human beings) on entering a surgery, a ward or an office. This applies to patients and staff alike; therefore these form a core within the specifics of the defined area, in which there are issues that the average citizen would not encounter on a regular basis. Implementation of the NHS and Community Care Act 1990 could well create a less obvious definition between medical and business ethics in some areas. The change within the NHS means that instead of being one large multifacetted service, it will comprise a number of purchasers and providers working on behalf of the consumer (previously known as the patient or client). Business strategies will be involved and therefore medical and business ethics could become entangled in some areas.

The following example indicates the distinctions between these three forms of theorizing.

> A shopkeeper discovers that a seven-year-old boy has stolen a packet of sweets, considering this to be 'bad' behaviour and therefore unacceptable. The shopkeeper then has to decide whether the child should be chastised with no further action, whether the child's parents should be informed for them to be aware of the misdemeanour and deal with it themselves, or whether the police should be involved as this is a juvenile crime.

• This is practical ethics, where the situation is happening—a decision must be made (*practical ethics*).

• Reference to the shopkeeper's moral principles, values or theory could determine any decision about what action to take. For example, if the shopkeeper feels that it is wrong to steal and all cases of stealing should be punished, then the matter may well be referred to the police (*ethical/moral theory*).

• This is the part which—rather than help the shopkeeper decide on a course of action—would consider what was meant by 'bad' behaviour or 'crime' (*meta-ethics*).

WHAT IS A MORAL ISSUE?

According to the *Concise Oxford Dictionary* (1988), an 'issue' is a 'point in question' or 'an important topic for discussion'. Similarly, *The Dictionary of Philosophy and Psychology* (Baldwin, 1960) defines an issue as 'a topic of discussion or controversy'. It would probably be fair to say that an issue is an important topic on which the majority of people will have an opinion. Opinions will vary—otherwise there is no real issue—and may be based on different values and beliefs; it is this variance that leads to dilemmas.

Peter Singer in *Practical Ethics* (1979) points out that, contrary to popular opinion, morals are not to do with sexual prohibition, rather they are more concerned with the rights and wrongs of everyday life. So what is a *moral issue*? It would appear to be an important topic relating to the rights and wrongs of everyday living, for example, the value placed on life—this would involve routine dealings with other people, views on capital punishment, etc.; it could also relate to extraordinary events that occur, the Gulf War for example.

Many problems have an obvious moral dimension, some reveal moral issues on closer inspection. However, Johnson (1990) warns of the possibility of people, once aware of medical ethics, analysing every *clinical* decision for moral issues; some might call this 'over-ethicizing'. It is also his opinion that confusion arises between ethics and etiquette, in that social convention can be mistaken for moral principle, indeed it has been suggested that until fairly recently the majority of doctors felt that medical ethics as a subject dealt primarily with issues of professional etiquette. He gives as an example the practice of patients only being referred to consultants by a general practitioner (GP)—failure to comply with this practice is against etiquette not ethics. Many people hope that this practice regarding referrals will be changed in the future, as the *Winterton Report* (1992) suggests that there should be direct referral opportunities for midwives.

WHAT IS A MORAL DILEMMA?

Campbell (1984) describes a moral dilemma as a situation where:

> ... one is faced with two alternative choices, neither of which seems a satisfactory solution to the problem.

This is accepted by others, including Johnson (1990), who qualifies it further by stating that the alternatives are 'apparently equal'. In a way, encountering a dilemma could be considered similar to facing crossroads, or a forked road, with inadequate directions:

A driver has some idea of where he wants to get to, he would also like to arrive in the quickest time but with least hazards on the way. In the absence of a map, written instructions or adequate signposting he has to make a decision—but will it be the right one?

Obviously, the result in this situation is not so crucial as one involving the treatment of a person—be it medical or social treatment. The example given is not a moral dilemma, it is merely a simplified indication of the basic problem. The shopkeeper in the earlier example could be seen to be in a similar situation with three possible routes to follow.

The moral dilemmas that midwives face may not be any greater than those faced by others, just different. They are governed professionally by the UKCC. Their *Code of Professional Conduct* (1992) for those professions mentioned, states, in the first two of 16 points:

> As a registered nurse, midwife or health visitor, you are personally accountable for your practice and, in the exercise of your professional accountability, must:

1. ... act always in such a manner as to promote and safeguard the inter-
   ests and well-being of patients and clients;

2. ... ensure that no action or omission *on your part, or within your*
   sphere of responsibility, is detrimental to the interests, condition or
   safety of patients and clients.

Even considering situations in which one might have to take account of these
two moral requirements indicates the real possibility of dilemmas emerging. An
example of a moral dilemma faced by midwives could be as follows.

A primiparous woman is admitted in established labour. She has a birthplan
that states that under no circumstances will she give consent to an episiotomy.
During the second stage of labour progress is slow but positive, however, the
perineum remains thick and rigid. This is explained to the woman but she
maintains her position regarding episiotomy. As time progresses the fetal
heart shows signs of slight distress, to the point where most midwives would
consider episiotomy to be the action of choice, but still the woman withholds
consent. The midwife could either continue and hope that the fetus will
survive—obviously notifying appropriate personnel—or she could perform
the procedure without consent in order to protect the fetus. If she carries out
the episiotomy without consent she could face a claim of battery against her.
Neither is the ideal solution. This is further complicated by a British court
decision in 1992 to overrule a mother's wishes in favour of her fetus
(Dimond, 1993). (Maternal versus fetal rights is discussed in Chapter 6.)

It is not only in situations such as this, however, that moral dilemmas occur.
Imagine yourself as the central figure in the next example.

Jenny has passed her driving test and has an old car in which she and her
three flatmates travel to their college. She and her friends have acquired tick-
ets for a particular idol's concert in London. The group cannot afford the
train fare but, if Jenny is prepared to drive, they can afford the petrol
between them. Jenny agrees to this. On the morning of the concert, as they
are preparing to leave, Jenny receives a telephone call from her mother to say
that her grandmother has been taken to hospital and is seriously ill.

In Jenny's place what do you do? Do you go to the hospital and thereby break a
promise and disappoint your friends who were relying on you, or do you continue on the outing and neglect your grandmother and parents?

The examples that have been used should indicate that not only are dilemmas created by more than one possible course of action, but they often also deal
in hypotheticals by the fact that actual consequences cannot be predicted accurately, merely supposed. If the outcomes are certain there is no initial dilemma.
Beauchamp and Childress (1989) describe two forms of moral dilemma: one form

is where there seems good reason to support both performing and not performing a particular act, as in the case of the woman who refused the episiotomy;
the other is where the particular action is considered by some to be right and by
others to be wrong. This would include cases such as a woman—with a known
abnormal fetus—making a decision regarding abortion. They also indicate that
not all philosophers accept that moral dilemmas exist; these philosophers are
monist—believing that all actions should be governed by one supreme duty,
'good will' for example. Immanuel Kant was one such person, believing that all
actions should be performed out of a sense of duty and right reason, never
through inclination. He believed that the *intended* results of an action were to
be judged rather than the *actual* results, hence the moral dilemma regarding the
outcome of chosen actions does not exist (Norman, 1988).

WHAT IS A MORAL CONFLICT?

On first consideration it could be assumed that conflict and dilemma are roughly
the same. However, Beauchamp and Childress (1989) make it clear that it is
actually the *conflict* between moral principles or obligations that often causes
the *dilemmas*. Johnson (1990) agrees with this and indicates two types of such
conflict, one being the conflict within a principle—he uses autonomy as an
example. Even if we accept autonomy as a moral value that should be promoted
and protected, whose is most important? That of the midwife or the client? The
second type is where two separate principles conflict, here we can consider
again our previous case of the labouring woman refusing an episiotomy which
could protect her baby; the midwife has an obligation to value the life of the
fetus but also to consider the interests and well-being of the woman.

It is important to remember that although everyone comes into contact with
health professionals at least once in their lives, they do not all work within this
sphere. It may therefore be useful to consider the moral conflicts that people
might face outside their working lives. They could include what a young
adolescent experiences when he becomes worried about a friend's apparent
addiction to drugs.

Until he became worried, the adolescent probably felt that no dilemma existed, at least with regard to his friend. The fact that he is worried indicates that he would like to do something about it, but what? He has two basic choices, each with different consequences:

CHOICE 1
Do nothing. Consider that the friend is experimenting with aspects of life in order to enable him to make the transition into a self-determining adult. Alternatively, he may consider that it is none of his business and he has no right to interfere.

CONSEQUENCES
• The friend soon decides that this is not for him and gets on with his life. (If it has reached the point where our subject is concerned then this is an unlikely outcome.)
• The friend becomes increasingly antisocial as a result of his addiction, possibly engaging in criminal activities to support his habit.

Or more dramatically...

• The friend dies from continued drug abuse—either by developing disease(s) through his lifestyle or by overdosing or using 'unclean' drugs.

CHOICE 2
Tell his parents, in order that advice can be sought in time.

CONSEQUENCES
• The friend is furious at the breach in 'friendship' (i.e. confidentiality). He continues to use drugs but has nothing more to do with the 'sneak'. Our subject is not only without his best friend, he is no longer on hand to care for him and get help if needed.
• After the initial trauma of being 'found out' by his parents, the lad is thankful that his friend sought help for him in time.

This situation highlights that neither of the choices can be considered completely satisfactory, hence the adolescent's dilemma. Basically should he do nothing and lose his friend, either to a traumatic lifestyle or even through death, or should he take action and lose his friend through betrayal of trust? Either way it would appear that he will lose out.

Hopefully it is obvious that moral conflicts and dilemmas occur in every-day life, not just in specific areas like medicine and midwifery. As previously stated, they are situations of uncertainty in which people find themselves facing choices; the more difficult it is to predict the consequences of an action, the greater the dilemma (Campbell, 1984). In 'Jenny's' situation (p.19), perhaps compromise is possible—a visit to see the grandmother on the way to London. Compromise, however, is not always possible. How do you compromise between life or death when your choice of actions may lead to one or the other result?

HOW DO WE RESOLVE THE CONFLICTS—DO WE NEED ETHICAL THEORIES?

It was stated earlier that ethical theory is intended to create a mechanism with which to solve our moral problems, but is it needed? People with no back-ground in the study of ethics also have to make their decisions. Some everyday decisions would appear to be made intuitively or practically, some with a great deal of 'heart-searching', according to personal beliefs and values. It could be suggested that very little formal, ethical theorizing occurs. Generally, people would state that it is a matter of instinct, intuition or conscience and, for some, that it is dependent on circumstances. When it comes to the decision-making of a midwife about a client, or a doctor about a patient, there are legal aspects to be considered. Those people determining the legalities will, no doubt, consult the theories; one should therefore have a basic understanding of what these are based on.

The variety of theories that have been developed indicate the fact that philosophers cannot agree which is the most appropriate. In fact some, the sub-jectivists, would suggest that theories are unnecessary. They say that, as beliefs about morality cannot be true or false, there is no way of determining a correct way of living or acting, therefore no mechanism can be constructed (Norman, 1988). Norman later quotes Bertrand Russell as stating that when two people disagree about values, there is no difference in objective truths, merely a differ-ence in taste. He explains that Ayer and Stevenson developed Russell's view into a theory known as 'emotivism' where feelings and attitudes play a part, as opposed to 'descriptivism' which is based on facts.

Traditionally, two major theories are considered and these will therefore be outlined. The author would then like to consider the possibility of an alternative.

ETHICAL THEORIES

Utilitarianism and deontology are considered to be rival theories in moral philosophy.

UTILITARIANISM

Utilitarianism is an ethical theory that claims to be based on the only appropriate interpretation of human nature available to philosophy. All human beings (and animals) have one thing in common—they seek pleasure and avoid pain. Individuals therefore pursue those activities that will, in the end, at least bring them pleasure and avoid those that will cause them pain. If this is true of all individuals, then a moral individual should have regard not only for their own pleasures and pains but also those of others. When making choices they should seek to maximize pleasure and minimize pain for all involved. Thus the general principle on which utilitarianism is based is that a moral action is that which creates the 'greatest happiness' for the greatest number. This has a certain appeal at a basic level because, as Glover (1988) tells us, whether we are utilitarian or not, most of us take some account of the probable effects of our actions on others but a number of criticisms can be raised. However, before considering these, it is necessary to distinguish between the two forms of utilitarianism available: act-utilitarianism and rule-utilitarianism.

Act-utilitarianism

This is the classic or traditional form supported and developed, for instance, by Bentham, Mill and Sidgwick in the 18th and 19th centuries. In this form of utilitarianism, every single action is judged by its consequences.

The principle is simple and easy to grasp as every action is assessed in terms of the happiness it will produce: the greater the degree of happiness, benefit or good, the greater the chance that the act was right. It is a method of seeking answers to questions in an objectively calculable way, the only acceptable solutions being those that create maximum good. Efficiency is often sought by decision makers and act-utilitarianism can provide this too, in that conflicting interests can be compared and assessed in terms of their capacity for producing good.

Rule-utilitarianism

This modification of act-utilitarianism assesses an act according to moral rules, the right rule being that which would produce the maximum 'good'. Therefore, instead of individual actions being assessed according to the principle of utility, they are assessed according to moral rules of conduct to enable them to comply with the principle of utility. This means that an act is right if it falls under the right rule—the rule is right if general observance of it would maximize utility. Let us look at this in everyday terms:

> It is customary for British Gas to send out quarterly bills to their consumers. At the end of the summer quarter, the occupants of a particular household received a bill for 10p. This is because they only use gas for central heating and had not required the service during that quarter. They complained that 'handling' charges would be far in excess of the amount due, suggesting that their bill should be half-yearly or yearly.

In a large organization such as this, there needs to be streamlining of certain procedures, hence the computerized sending of all bills at the same time. In order to fulfil this family's request, it would mean changing the whole system. This in itself may not appear to be a problem but how often would it occur that such small bills would be received? In fact, changing the system would probably create hardship for many people as this would entail paying much larger bills, albeit less frequently. It would appear to be more sensible, in this case, to maintain the rule of quarterly charges (despite the few anomalies) rather than create greater problems by changing the rule to suit the few. There is the need to determine the consequential differences in order to determine the validity of the rules but with caution to prevent the rules from becoming too specific, and therefore ridiculous, or in fact creating a slide-back to the act itself.

Some criticisms of utilitarianism

It is necessary to consider whether the claims on behalf of utilitarianism are justified. It is considered to be simple and calculable in terms of utility, forward-looking to the *possible* benefits and *probable* costs. However, the apparent simplicity of assessing everything in terms of happiness or good disappears when one closely examines happiness itself. What is 'happiness' or 'pleasure' and how does one measure utility or usefulness? It is possible that everyone would have a concept of these words but would they have the same concepts and the same priorities? When considering the 'greatest happiness' principle, it is difficult to assess whether this is achieved by creating a lot of happiness for a few people or a little for a greater number of people.

It is also preferable to know whose utility should be considered. People would presumably start with themselves but then would also need to consider their families, as individuals can have a major effect on each other's lives.

People also affect—or are affected by—those they work with, those they live near, and the nation of which they are a part; if happiness is to be maximized, very soon people could justify personal responsibility for the world. How should the happiness of different people(s) be compared? Traditionalists view happiness as a mental state but surely this can vary in quality and quantity. Glover (1988) asks:

What is there in common between the mental state experienced during a happy picnic and that experienced when your child is born?

As he rightly says 'The problems are obvious'. Total happiness could mean increasing the levels of pleasure of existing people, or it could be increasing numbers of happy people. If increasing numbers means increasing the size of the nation/population then this could cause a decrease in the level of individual happiness by overcrowding, inadequate food, poor health and therefore increased mortality and morbidity rates. Some, including Bentham, say that animals should be included, but even if considerations are restricted to human beings, which generations matter? When contemplating the happiness of future generations, it is not certain what life will be like for them and, therefore, it is not possible to anticipate their pleasure accurately.

Utilitarianism can place unreasonable demands on individuals, considering everyone as equal when clearly they are often unequal, particularly with regard to responsibility. A woman with children would be considered to have different responsibilities to a woman with no dependants, whereas someone whose job includes policy making has responsibility for the greatest good for an even greater number of people. Also, while considering communitarian outcomes, the individual may be required to sacrifice personal happiness in favour of the majority. There are moral objections to consequentialism in that the 'means' may include acts of dishonesty, injustice and so on. For non-utilitarians such acts would be against their codes of conduct as this could mean that 'local' misery is created in order to achieve 'global' pleasure. This can create conflicts with individual integrity and has little regard for the protection of individuals. Take, for example, the following situation from Smart and Williams (1988)—it is not a midwifery situation but one that highlights the difference between the utilitarian and the deontologist:

Jim is a botanist on an expedition in South America. He finds himself in a small town where 20 Indians are tied up ready for execution, following acts of protest against the government. The captain, Pedro, having explained the situation, offers Jim a guest's privilege of killing one of the Indians himself. If he accepts, as a special mark of the occasion, the other Indians will be freed. If he refuses, then there is no special occasion and Pedro will have them all killed as previously planned.

If Jim is a utilitarian he will have no qualms about carrying out the execution—after all, to lose one life in order to save 19 produces a better consequence than losing all 20 lives. If he is a non-consequentialist then the possibility of committing murder, regardless of the consequences, would be against his moral integrity. If Jim killed the one, then he would be responsible for that one death. However, what would his responsibility be if Pedro carried out the 20 executions? Would he be responsible for the deaths of the other 19? This would be negative responsibility which a utilitarian may well consider appropriate in this case, although a non-utilitarian would not accept this, accepting only that Jim is responsible for his own actions.

There can be definite practical problems with utilitarianism—the difficulty of predicting all the possible consequences of an action, and difficulty in accurate prediction of those considered. How—in fact—are the consequences planned for? What time span is considered? How broad is the thinking and how many alternatives are to be considered? If we are seeking to arrive at a decision then there is often no time for protracted pondering.

DEONTOLOGY

Deon is the Greek word for duty, and, as the term suggests, deontological theory considers duty to be the central issue, as opposed to teleological considerations of deontology, which say that everything has been created by God to serve mankind. Deontologists believe that what is good in the world stems from people doing their duty. They consider duty first, regardless of the consequences, with the notion of happiness fitting in where, and if, it can. Perhaps this can be illustrated by considering the men who—despite personal risk to themselves and the knowledge that they may never return to their families—enrolled in the armed forces in the two World Wars. Whether we approve of armed conflict or not, we must assume that at least some of those who did not wait to be conscripted did so from a sense of duty. This duty was essentially to 'King and Country' and in the defence of their own families.

As with utilitarianism, there is more than one theoretical version in deontology; in fact there are three. These theories not only compete with utilitarianism but also with each other.

Rational monism

This moral theory was constructed by Immanuel Kant who claimed not to be creating a radically new moral theory, rather he thought he was formalizing how people already thought. In his view, the only moral actions are those performed through a sense of duty. One's duty is to do what is rational and moral, all actions proceeding from a 'good will' will be moral in this sense. To help identify which actions are—or more properly which *are not* moral—he offered his theory of the 'categorical imperative'. This is about 'oughts' and 'ought nots', very definite and decisive: duty for duty's sake. The hypothetical imperative, on the other hand, is less definite, using terms such as 'if ... then', 'in order to ...', 'if you want to do or achieve X then do Y' or 'in order to achieve X do Y'. For Kant this was not definite enough. His first moral test of an action was by universalizability:

Act only on that maxim through which you can at the same time will that it should become a universal law.

(Kant, in Paton, 1981)

His second test involved the consideration of the autonomy of people:

Act in such a way that you always treat humanity, whether in your own person or in the person of any other, never simply as a means, but always at the same time as an end.

(Kant, in Paton, 1981)

This has been presented very simply by Gillon (1986). He explains Kant's argument as follows:

Kant believed that the truth of his moral theory was a necessary consequence of the rational nature of human beings. He believed that he could prove that any rational being necessarily recognised himself to be bound by what Kant called the 'supreme moral law'. [...]

This supreme moral law stemmed from the fact that rational agents (or persons) intrinsically possessed an absolute moral value (in contrast with inanimate objects and 'beasts'), which rendered them members of what he called the kingdom of 'ends in themselves'. Not only did all rational agents recognise themselves as ends in themselves but, in so far as they were rational, they also recognised all other rational agents to be ends in themselves, who should be respected as such.

These two examples may help to see this law more practically:

I keep my promises. If everybody did, would it be right?

Clearly, in this case, it would (depending on the promises), but:

I do not agree with paying National Insurance payments, therefore I shall refuse to pay them. If everyone refused to pay, would it be right?

In this case, regardless of personal views about this charge, it would not be right as there would be no money for the provision of services, irrespective of the fact that this brings us into the realms of criminal law.

Doctors are expected to be deontological in that that they are expected to abide by the Laws of Humanity as formulated by the Declaration of Geneva. Similar expectations of nurses, midwives and health visitors are held, as determined by the UKCC in the *Code of Professional Conduct* (1992) and the *Midwife's Code of Practice* (1991). These are not scientific laws, nor are they positive laws of which a legal system is comprised, rather they are natural or moral laws.

'Traditional' deontology

This has a strong religious basis, with a belief in God and the sanctity of life. Moral duties are taken from the Ten Commandments and it would seem logical to assume that devout Christians, and those other beliefs where the Commandments in general—and the sanctity of life in particular—are featured, would consider this theory to be the basis of their moral decision making. As can be seen, the Ten Commandments form a good basic model of 'dos and don'ts' and do not create moral conflicts. The avoidance of conflict occurs because each addresses a different prohibition or obligation, therefore it is possible to abide by them all simultaneously.

> *Thou shalt have none other Gods before me.*
> *Thou shalt not make thee any graven image.*
> *Thou shalt not take the name of the Lord thy God in vain.*
> *Keep the sabbath day to sanctify it.*
> *Honour thy father and thy mother.*
> *Thou shalt not kill.*
> *Neither shalt thou commit adultery.*
> *Neither shalt thou steal.*
> *Neither shalt thou bear false witness.*
> *Neither shalt thou desire thy neighbour's wife.*
>
> The Holy Bible

Intuitionistic pluralism

Unlike rational monism, this version of deontology advocates no supreme principle, rather it suggests that there are several moral rules or obligations to be followed that are of equal importance.

There is always the possibility of rule conflict though, so how is this resolved? Ross considered seven prima-facie duties which he believed 'any reflective person would intuitively accept' (Gillon, 1986), and these were to be carried out unless specific situations proved prohibitive:

1. DUTY OF FIDELITY This involves keeping promises, being loyal and not deceiving. Is this what we expect of our Government as well as individuals?

2. DUTY OF BENEFICENCE The obligation to help others.

3. DUTY OF NON-MALEFICENCE Not harming others; this, says Gillon (1986), is more stringent than the previous duty.

4. DUTY OF JUSTICE To ensure fair play.

5. DUTY OF REPARATION An obligation to make amends.

6. DUTY OF GRATITUDE To repay in some way those who have helped us (owed to special people such as parents); this also includes loyalty.

7. DUTY OF SELF-IMPROVEMENT.

The problems arise when these duties also conflict, for instance, in order to keep a promise or be loyal to a friend you have to be disloyal to or offend a parent—here there is conflict between the duties of fidelity and gratitude. As no one duty has an automatic lead, there is no hierarchy. So how do people decide how and when to override one duty by another? In the Jewish and Roman Catholic religions, in Kant's view and to some extent in the British legal system, there is a system whereby such conflicts are resolved—it is called 'casuistry'. This system allows for disentanglement of the conflicting rules and reordering them in accordance with the situation. Despite the pitfalls created by conflict of duties, it is interesting to note that medical ethics has found this model attractive. For midwives it is apparent in the UKCC's *Code of Professional Conduct* (1992). Arguably the most common problem arising for midwives, from the 16 'duties' laid down in the *Code*, is the conflict of autonomy:

1. Act always in such a manner as to promote and safeguard the interests and well-being of patients and clients; [...]
6. Work in a collaborative and co-operative manner with health care professionals and others involved in providing care, and recognise and respect their particular contributions within the care team.

The problem that arises usually involves conflict between the autonomy of the woman and that of the midwife, but also between the midwife and other health care professionals (see 'Autonomy and consent').

Another alternative?

It was stated earlier (p.16) that some philosophers—particularists—reject the need for formal theories which can then be applied to every situation. They prefer to develop the moral sensibilities of individuals, enabling them to discern the rights and wrongs as they arise and act with the flexibility required of the specific situation. The principle of truth-telling may be a good example here. If, according to deontological belief, one has a duty to tell the truth at all times, what happens on the occasions when telling the truth will cause offence? If to tell a lie would create no harm, but would prevent causing offence, that could be a better course of action—without having to mentally conduct a utilitarian experiment to see which course produced the greatest amount of good.

Particularism gives this flexibility (McNaughton, 1988). It does not say that we can ignore morality, rather that we educate children through all the avenues of socialization, to recognize the right action to take for the situation in which they find themselves. This education would undoubtedly change its style and content according to the age and development of the child. Some moral guidance would be offered in the form of commands to a young child, as a means of protection, until the child is mature enough to be discerning.

From the midwifery point of view, an 'avenue of socialization' could be the inclusion of moral rights and principles in the educational programme—which should then be applied in practice—while ignoring the traditional duty-based and consequentialist theories.

SUGGESTED READING

Beauchamp, T.L. and Childress, J.F. (1989) *Principles of Biomedical Ethics*, 3rd edn, Oxford University Press, Oxford, Chapter 2.

Gillon, R. (1986) *Philosophical Medical Ethics*, John Wiley and Sons, Chichester, Chapters 3, 4 and 5.

Glover, J. (1988) *Causing Death and Saving Lives*, John Wiley and Sons, Chichester, Chapter 4.

Johnson, A.G. (1990) *Pathways in Medical Ethics*, Edward Arnold, London.

Smart, J.J.C. and Williams, B. (1988) *Utilitarianism For and Against*, Cambridge University Press, Cambridge.

REFERENCES

Entries marked '*' are bibliographical entries rather than—or as well as—references.

*Aristotle, *Ethics* (ed. and trans. J. Warrington, 1975), Dent, London.

Baldwin, J.M. (1960) *Dictionary of Philosophy and Psychology Volume 1*, Peter Smith, Massachusetts, USA, p.576.

*Beauchamp, T.L. and Childress, J.F. (1989) *Principles of Biomedical Ethics*, 3rd edn, Oxford University Press, Oxford, pp.4–5, 35.

*Campbell, A.V. (1984) *Moral Dilemmas in Medicine*, 3rd edn, Churchill Livingstone, London, p.2.

Concise Oxford Dictionary (1988) (ed. R.E. Allen), Clarendon Press, Oxford.

*Dimond, B. (1993) Client autonomy and choices. *Modern Midwife*, **3**(1), 15–16.

*Gillon, R. (1986) *Philosophical Medical Ethics*, John Wiley and Sons, Chichester, p.18.

*Glover, J. (1988) *Causing Death and Saving Lives*, John Wiley and Sons, Chichester, Chapter 4, p.63.

HMSO (1990) *NHS and Community Care Act 1990*, HMSO, London.

Holy Bible, Collins, London, Genesis, 5: 7–21.

*Jenkins, R.and Murphy, A. (1991) *Accountability, the Law and the Midwife*, DLC, South Bank University, London.

*Johnson, A.G. (1990) *Pathways in Medical Ethics*, Edward Arnold, London, pp.28–29, 33.

Kant, I., In *The Moral Law* (ed. H.J. Paton, 1981), The Anchor Press, Essex.

*McNaughton, D. (1988) *Moral Vision*, Blackwell, Oxford, pp.200–203.

*Norman, R. (1988) *The Moral Philosophers*, Clarendon Press, Oxford, pp.1–2, 3, 98, 226–227.

*Rumbold, R. (1991) *Ethics in Nursing and Midwifery Practice*, DLC, South Bank University, London.

*Singer, P. (1989) *Practical Ethics*, Cambridge University Press, Cambridge, pp.2, 13.

*Smart, J.J.C. and Williams, B. (1988) *Utilitarianism For and Against*, Cambridge University Press, Cambridge, pp.98–99.

UKCC (1991) *A Midwife's Code of Practice*.

UKCC (1992) *Code of Professional Conduct for the Nurse, Midwife and Health Visitor*, 2nd edn.

*Warnock, G.J. (1967) *Contemporary Moral Philosophy*, Macmillan, London.

Winterton, N. (1992) *House of Commons' Health Committee's Second Report: Maternity Services, Volume 1*, HMSO, London.

PART TWO

CASE STUDIES

1.

INTRODUCTION

It is important to consider and avoid, with all the cases and questions, the temptation to say 'It depends' or 'It's up to her/him or them' (Downie and Calman, 1987). This may occur particularly when people feel threatened and do not want to face or expose their feelings on certain subjects, especially if it is a topic that they have never openly discussed before. It is also important, while acknowledging the earlier warning against over-ethicizing, to avoid a tendency to fall back on clinical as opposed to ethical distinctions. This situation can be seen in midwifery practice with regard to the rupturing of fetal membranes in labour; midwives can often be heard to extol the virtues of leaving them intact, their reasoning, however, is usually clinically based rather than on the grounds of the woman's autonomy (see the case study 'Autonomy and consent', pp.59–76). If the reader wishes to use these case studies with her peers, she must remember the need for a safe environment when people are expected to expose their views; she may wish to involve a tutor to facilitate the group in setting up this safety. It needs to be stated at the outset that everyone is entitled to their own opinions and that there may be considerable differences within the group, but also that it would be expected that there should be an honest conflict of views. Obviously sensitivity is required as some participants may well have experienced some of the situations under discussion; it is also necessary to prevent the formation of 'encounter' groups. Facilitation may also be required in order to tease out areas that have been overlooked or avoided; someone may be required to play 'Devil's advocate' in order to achieve this.

The following chapters include six case studies dealing with topics about which midwives have expressed concern (to the author): confidentiality; accountability; autonomy and consent; screening for fetal abnormality; maternal rights versus fetal rights; and resource allocation. The case studies have been constructed to be of particular interest to midwives of all levels, including situations that can and do occur. For those with a deeper understanding of medical ethics, seemingly unrelated cases create fewer problems; they are better equipped to apply the principles to various situations. There may be many, however, who enter midwifery without such depth of understanding. It may therefore be preferable to apply the principles within the sphere of midwifery practice before developing the ability of application in other fields.

The first two case studies consider the midwife and her actions, whereas the third involves her with another health professional, in this case it happens to be a doctor. Cases four and five do not focus on dilemmas specific to a midwife but they are situations in which midwives have a responsibility—they should know something of the ethics that are involved. The last case involves resource allocation, allocation at a level that would not directly involve a midwife. However, midwives do have opinions regarding the use of limited resources and they should, therefore, have some idea of the possible processes involved in the decision-making: some of them may become senior managers and their input would then be required.

As previously stated, the characters in the case studies, and other examples used are not intended to depict any particular race or social class—names were selected at random. To consider different races, religions or social classes could possibly add a new dimension to the cases; this could be carried through by interested readers if they wished to consider what difference, if any, it would make.

Each case study is accompanied by the theory relating to the major issues expected to be raised. Where appropriate technical information has also been incorporated; this appears in 'Further discussion'. During consideration of the questions, particularly during any group discussion, it is quite possible that other moral issues and philosophical principles may arise; this has been anticipated to a certain extent by bringing some of the other points into 'Further discussion' and, where applicable, indication is given to which other chapter may be useful. However, to discuss all principles that arise would make some chapters too complex; the reader may wish to note those that arise and are not dealt with, in order to pursue them further.

If the ethics module of the reader's course is to be assessed, then written work could be practised around the cases, perhaps using the questions as a basis for formulating an answer plan. This may encourage additional reading including the consideration of newspaper articles, women's magazines and television programmes, not only 'known texts'. This may well indicate the tendency for one-sided views to be reported by the media.

REFERENCES

These references can all be considered as bibliographical entries.

Burnard, P. and Chapman, C.M. (1988) *Professional and Ethical Issues in Nursing*, John Wiley and Sons, Chichester.

Curzon, L.B. (1985) *Teaching in Further Education*, 3rd edn, Cassell Educational, London, pp.215–218.

Downie, R.S. and Calman, K.C. (1987) *Healthy Respect—Ethics in Health Care*, Faber and Faber, London, p.140.

Gillon, R. (1990) Teaching Medical Ethics: Impressions from the USA, in *Medicine, Medical Ethics and the Value of Life* (ed. P. Byrne), John Wiley and Sons, Chichester.

Jenkins, R. and Murphy, A. (1991) *Accountability, the Law and the Midwife*, DLC, South Bank University, London.

Pyne, R.H. (1981) *Professional Discipline in Nursing*, Blackwell Scientific Publications, Oxford.

RCM (1989) *Practical Guidance for Midwives Facing Ethical or Moral Dilemmas*, London.

Rowson, R. (1992) Ethics and care, Part 1: Making judgements (Open Learning Programme). *Nursing Times* , **88**(24), i–viii.

Rumbold, R. (1991) *Ethics in Nursing and Midwifery Practice*, DLC, South Bank University, London.

Thompson, A. (1989) Conflict and Covenant—Ethics in the Midwifery Curriculum. *Midwives Chronicle*, June, 191–197.

2.

CONFIDENTIALITY

CASE STUDY

Hannah was expecting her third baby and was hoping for a DOMINO delivery. This was mainly so that she did not have to leave her daughters—Naomi who was four years old and Carmel who was two—for longer than was necessary.

At 34 weeks' gestation, however, she was admitted to the consultant unit with a moderate, painless antepartum haemorrhage. Following an ultrasound scan, the diagnosis of grade 3 placenta praevia was made and Hannah was advised that she would need to remain in hospital. During the admission procedure the midwife, Cobi, explained that Hannah would remain in hospital until delivery. She explained that this would be by caesarean section at around 38 weeks, unless circumstances demanded earlier intervention. Hannah became very distressed and said that she could not stay in hospital even though she understood the risks to herself and her baby.

Cobi eventually persuaded Hannah to calm down and gently probed for the reason for such agitation about admission; she anticipated a fear of hospitals, perhaps based on a previous bad experience. Eventually Hannah explained, having first secured a promise from Cobi that she would not repeat any of what she would hear. Hannah felt that she could not stay in hospital because her husband would sexually abuse the two little girls if she was not there to protect them. He had apparently abused them before but she was usually able to prevent it—so long as she was there. This was also her reason for requesting a DOMINO delivery.

Cobi tried to persuade Hannah that she should see a social worker, for the sake of the children and in order to get some help for her husband. Hannah would not agree to this as she remembered the situations that occurred in Cleveland, UK. She also forbade Cobi from seeking help on her behalf, on the grounds that she had spoken in the strictest confidence. It was a difficult situation for Cobi; however, after careful thought she decided that she could not breach confidentiality. She told the Registrar that Hannah would discharge herself if they insisted on keeping her. The Registrar would not take the responsibility for discharging Hannah with a placenta praevia, therefore she discharged herself. Cobi contacted the community midwives and they agreed to visit twice daily in order to listen to the fetal heart and observe any blood loss; they were not given the reason for her self-discharge. Cobi wondered what would happen following the caesarean section.

Following a number of small haemorrhages, Hannah started labouring at 37 weeks. An emergency caesarean section was performed and Hannah discharged herself and her son two days later, with no explanation other than wanting to be at home with her daughters .

QUESTIONS FOR CONSIDERATION BY THE READER

1. Why is confidentiality an important principle?

2. Was Cobi only accountable to Hannah for maintaining confidentiality?

3. Did Cobi have any duty to the children – Naomi and Carmel?

4. Is there ever a time when it is acceptable to breach confidentiality?

5. What would have been the likely outcome if Cobi had disclosed the information?

An issue that is not discussed here, but which readers may wish to pursue, is child abuse.

Question 1. Why is confidentiality an important principle?

In order to determine the importance of maintaining confidentiality, it is necessary to consider what it means. Many definitions are very wordy but they almost all contain the word 'trust'. Relationships in midwifery, as in all areas of health care, are centred on trust. A woman entrusts a midwife with a great deal of personal and generally private information. When she does this she has the right to expect that this information will remain confidential, being passed on only with her consent. Her right in this case is a moral one as there is no statutory right to confidentiality (Mason and McCall Smith, 1987). A breach of confidentiality can lead to legal action in the civil courts; it can also lead to criminal action but this is not for the breach itself, rather it is for the use to which the information is put and the harm that ensues.

In the case of midwifery/medical records, however, it is not considered reasonable to seek specific consent for the passage of information between professionals caring for each woman/patient. This is covered by 'implied consent' (see the case study 'Autonomy and consent') where, in giving information that is to be recorded in the woman's/patient's file, the person is implying consent for other health care professionals who will have contact with her/him to have access to this information. This, however, is considered to be on a 'need to know' basis in that only those professionals who need to know the information – in order to care for the individual concerned – will be given access to it.

Consider the ward reporting system in your unit at the shift handover: Who is present? What information is passed on? Do all those people need to know all that information?

It could be suggested that this is one area where midwives fall down on the observance of the 'need to know' principle and, therefore, on the observance of confidentiality.

Question 2. Was Cobi only accountable to Hannah for maintaining confidentiality?

Hannah was not the only person to whom Cobi was accountable for maintaining confidentiality, although obviously she is the most important. Cobi is also accountable to her employer, through line management, for her actions. Professionally, she is accountable for her conduct to the UKCC, which also has a structure, starting with the Supervisor of Midwives. If she breaches confidentiality she is accountable in British civil law (not criminal law in this instance) should Hannah choose to make a claim against her. (For further consideration see the chapter 'Accountability'.)

Question 3. Did Cobi have any duty to the children— Naomi and Carmel?

Although generalizations can be unwise, it would probably be reasonable to suggest that most health care workers feel a responsibility for people in general, not just those in their care at any one time. Where health promotion and education are concerned this is acceptable but professionally Cobi's situation is more specific. Hannah is the client to whom Cobi owes a duty of care; there is no such duty owed to the two girls as they are not Cobi's clients/patients, even though midwives are concerned with family health and welfare.

Midwives are expected to 'serve the interests of society' (UKCC, 1992) added to which they are also members of the general public and as such may well be expected to consider the well-being of these children, regardless of the lack of duty of care. Society would appear to hold double standards regarding the actions of health care professionals; on the one hand expecting to take positive action in such circumstances, but on the other expecting the same professionals to uphold confidentiality. This is where the dilemma occurs (Finch, 1989). Apart from urging Hannah to disclose the information to an appropriate person, or at least allowing Cobi to do so, there are two basic options. Option one would be to alert the proper authorities that the girls may be in danger, thus breaching confidentiality—not an ideal solution. Option two would be to observe confidentiality and potentially leave the children at risk—again, not an ideal solution. Cobi must make her decision as a professional, however, not as a member of the public, as it was in this role that she received the information. She may have felt that she should approach her Supervisor of Midwives; from her own professional point of view this would be correct, but disclosing the information in this way is still breaching confidentiality (Silverton, 1992), especially if the Supervisor of Midwives decided to involve other agencies.

Question 4: Is there ever a time when it is acceptable to breach confidentiality?

Midwives, as with nurses and health visitors, are governed by the UKCC. Their booklet *Code of Professional Conduct* (1992), clause 10 states:

> *Protect all confidential information concerning patients and clients obtained in the course of professional practice and make disclosures only with consent, where required by the order of a court or where you can justify disclosure in the wider public interest.*

This is further explained in the booklet *Confidentiality* (UKCC, 1987), which is actually an expansion of the confidentiality clause (i.e. clause 9) as printed in the second edition of 'The Code' in 1984. As the booklet indicates, 'public interest' is interpreted as:

> *... the interests of an individual, of groups of individuals or society as a whole, and would encompass ... serious crime, child abuse and drug trafficking.*

It would appear that, under this clause, Cobi could have disclosed the information without being considered by the UKCC to be in breach of confidentiality (but Hannah would still be in a position to sue her). However, 'The Code' states that she must be able to 'justify disclosure ...'. It is possible that Cobi felt unable to justify it, in that she only had Hannah's word that abuse had occurred and that Hannah might not be telling the truth for some reason. Also, Cobi would need to tell Hannah that she was going to disclose the information and Hannah could then deny it. If this happened, the children would be no better off and there would probably be a breakdown of trust in Hannah's relationship with any midwife in the future.

Question 5: What would have been the likely outcome if Cobi had disclosed the information?

The possible outcomes are many and varied, partly dependent on Hannah's reaction to the disclosure of her allegation, but also on the manner of reaction by the relevant members of Social Services. Possibly the best result would include friends or local family being asked to care for the children during Hannah's hospitalization, perhaps giving the reason as being to help the father. Counselling of Hannah and her husband, together and separately, could take place calmly with appropriate help and support being started. The family could eventually be grateful to Cobi.

The worst situation would probably include a 'swoop' by Social Services to remove the children, Hannah discharging herself to go home to an angry and distressed husband, plus a civil law suit against Cobi for breach of confidentiality. Cobi could also be suspended from duty by her Supervisor of Midwives, ratified by the Local Supervising Authority, while awaiting investigation of her conduct.

It is obvious that a variety of situations could arise that would be between the best and the worst possibilities.

FURTHER DISCUSSION

(Note: The issue of child abuse will not be discussed here; it is a major, multi-facetted issue requiring far more than this book can offer.)

There are two terms that cover similar areas but which are considered to be separate—confidentiality and privacy—both of which can be infringed or breached.

Infringement of confidentiality

An infringement of X's confidentiality occurs only if the person to whom X disclosed the information in confidence, fails to protect that information or deliberately discloses it to someone without X's consent.

(Beauchamp and Childress, 1989)

To put this into context:

Shirley (the course tutor) tells Lorna (a colleague) that she is pregnant but that she does not want to tell anyone else as yet. If Lorna tells another colleague then this is deliberate disclosure. Also, Shirley's group of students could discuss with Lorna the fact that they are worried about Shirley as she looks pale, tired or ill. If Lorna, without thinking or because she did not want the students to be concerned unnecessarily, explained the reason for her colleague's appearance of ill-health then she is still guilty of the infringement of confidentiality.

Infringement of privacy

... only a person or institution to whom a patient grants information in a confidential relationship can be charged with violating confidentiality.

(Beauchamp and Childress, 1989)

For example:

If a person gains unauthorized access into a hospital records department or computer data bank, despite appropriate protections, this would be an infringement of privacy.

This situation is quite rare, but there are many everyday situations where confidentiality and/or privacy could be breached, as in the following example:

Midwife A conducts a 'booking interview' and the woman explains that she has previously had a termination of pregnancy (TOP) but that her partner does not know.

1. If midwife A discloses this information to the partner—by intention or accident—she is guilty of infringement of confidentiality.

2. If midwife B—perhaps at a later clinic or during labour—discloses information that she has read in the notes, she is also guilty of breaching confidentiality.

3. If midwife B were to leave the delivery room, having closed the case notes, and the partner opens them and reads part or all of the contents, perhaps out of passing interest rather than malice, then he is guilty of a breach of privacy.

4. If a situation occurred where the woman authorized the disclosure of information to her partner, the midwife is not guilty of any infringement, although, in effect, there is a loss of both confidentiality and privacy.

With regard to client's/patient's records, there are two acts with which readers should be familiar. The first is the *Data Protection Act 1984* (Sterling, 1984). This covers computer held records and therefore affects most hospitals in the UK; clients can apply to view recorded information regarding themselves. The second is the *Access to Health Records Act 1990* (HMSO, 1990), which came into force on 1 November 1991; clients are entitled to access to any written records made following this date. If they wish to access written records made prior to this date, they must make formal application but they may be refused.

In situations 1 and 2 above, the employing authority could also be accountable by vicarious liability as they hold a degree of responsibility for the actions of the staff in their employ (Mason and McCall Smith, 1987).

For whom is confidentiality/privacy important?

It is not difficult to remember that confidentiality should be maintained for all the women in our care. However, we must realize that sometimes relatives also choose to confide in us. The author has had a number of experiences where the health of the woman has been poor, with severe pre-eclampsia in repeated pregnancies, moderate-to-severe renal disease or repeated puerperal psychosis, where sterilization has been advised. In these particular cases it had been suggested that perhaps the partner could consider vasectomy rather than subject the woman to tubal ligation. In some of these cases the men confided that the partnerships were insecure and therefore future partnerships had to be considered. The consequences of breaching such confidences, from the viewpoint of the families concerned, would be devastating and, as professionals, we must not help to create such an outcome.

Another group to be considered are colleagues (at all levels). Apart from personal confidences that friends and colleagues may confide or exchange, there are occasions where it is possible to observe incidents or overhear conversations. This could involve a colleague being counselled for an error or oversight, or a problem occurring during a delivery. It would be an infringement of privacy to disclose this knowledge to another colleague, even if this was in support of the one with a problem.

The situation would be different, of course, if an incident was observed or overheard involving the probable act of misconduct of a member of staff; for instance, if there were apparent abuse of a woman or her baby, or an incident involving the administration of drugs, or evidence of drug/alcohol abuse by a member of staff. In any such situation, the observer should report the incident to her Supervisor of Midwives. The privacy of a member of staff cannot be considered above the welfare of the women and their babies in our care (UKCC, 1992, clause 13). The same would be the case with concerns regarding poor standards of care generally; this too should be reported to the Supervisor of Midwives and not to an outside agency, as this could be deemed a breach of the service's confidentiality and therefore a breach of contract.

When do health-care workers need to consider confidentiality?

There are many situations where care is required in the workplace. A woman's case notes—in whatever form—are obviously an area of concern, considering the amount and type of information recorded; it is important not to leave them available to onlookers or to allow other unauthorized access. This is an area where most midwives are probably very careful.

The 'report' conducted at a shift change, however, is not always considered with such concern. In some cases it occurs in a fairly public area of the ward or department, but even when greater privacy is sought it must be remembered that loud voices can travel through walls and down corridors. It is therefore possible for the woman being discussed, or any other woman or visitor, to overhear what is being said. Also, as previously stated, it could be that unnecessary information is given to staff who do not require it. The fact of a woman overhearing her own report is not particularly important in itself if she has been fully included in her own care. Problems arise if she feels other women could hear personal details about her, or if staff have been unprofessional by making unpleasant subjective comments about her.

The telephone is a wonderful invention (generally speaking) but to staff on a busy ward or delivery suite it can be the bane of their lives. It can also be a tool for breaching confidentiality, however innocently. It is very tempting to automatically answer questions over the telephone, rather than asking the woman what she would like said. For instance, it is a regular occurrence to have people asking if their friend or relative '...has had her baby yet, and if so, what did she have?'. It also seems to be a frequent occurrence that the caller is not the sister or mother-in-law that she claims to be, but a friend or neighbour. Christmas and New Year can create problems with the media (Johnson, 1990)—reporters from local press and television contact hospitals to determine whatever details they can regarding babies born on these occasions. Perhaps the worst of all is the estranged partner who, not admitting to the estrangement, asks 'Can you tell me if my wife/girlfriend has been admitted please? I have been trying to ring her from work, with no reply, and I am getting quite worried because she said she was not going out'. In all these situations it is so easy to answer, almost automatically, without really thinking of the consequences, especially during a very busy shift.

Meal breaks can be times when staff can be guilty of discussing many aspects of their work, including the 'interesting' or 'difficult' woman they were dealing with just before their break. This is not only failing to uphold the 'need to know' principle but the conversation could be overheard by the woman's relative or neighbour sitting at another table who also works at the hospital; also, some hospitals have visitors sharing the same facilities as the staff.

Applying theory to practice is an essential part of the education of students. There is really no better way than for you to discuss actual cases that you have been involved in, especially if you are particularly elated or distressed by the case (Osborne and Martin, 1989). However well you observe the anonymity rule, it is almost certain that another student will recognize the case from delivery suite, clinic or the neonatal unit. The author feels that students must have the benefit of such discussions, with the relief that often follows the discovery that someone else has also experienced such a situation. In order to do this, a room, possibly a classroom, should be designated a 'safe area' where discussions can take place freely but where the rule is that discussion finishes within that room, none of the information being discussed outside. Where assignment work is concerned, anonymity must always be observed; this is far easier because the work is prepared over a period of time, with time to think and plan properly, unlike the spontaneity experienced within a verbal discussion.

At the end of a working day or night it is hoped that the majority of staff go home to caring parents, partners, families or friends: people who are interested in what kind of day/night they have had. Possibly they have travelled home with colleagues on public transport, and perhaps they intend to go out for a meal with friends who find it fascinating to listen to tales of midwifery encounters. In all these situations it would be easy to relax and forget about confidentiality. To a great extent this is reasonable—midwives and other members of staff are not expected to be silent about their work, all that is required is that they maintain the confidentiality of the women/families in their care.

APPLYING THE THEORIES

A utilitarian view

By reporting the apparent situation, Hannah will be distressed, so will the husband initially, although he may eventually be relieved to get help. The midwife will also feel upset that she has had to breach confidentiality. However, on the positive side, the little girls will not suffer the abuse again, Hannah may remain in hospital to protect herself and her fetus from the risks of haemorrhage, and the midwife will know that she has acted to protect the children. The balance would appear to be in favour of reporting the abuse.

A deontological view

The midwife has a duty to Hannah, as her client, which rates more highly than a generalized duty to others in society. Her duty here would be to maintain confidentiality.

SUGGESTED READING CONCERNING CONFIDENTIALITY

Benjamin, M. and Curtis, J. (1986) *Ethics in Nursing*, 2nd edn, Oxford University Press, Oxford.
Carlisle, D. (1991) To tell or not to tell. *Nursing Times*, **87**(16), 46–47.
Department of Health (1992) *Child Protection—Guidance for Senior Nurses, Health Visitors and Midwives*, HMSO, London.
HMSO (1990) *Access to Health Records Act 1990*, HMSO, London.
Silverton, L. (1992) Confidence in cocaine. *MIDIRS Midwifery Digest*, **2**(2), 237–238.
Sterling, J.L. (1984) *Data Protection Act 1984—A guide to the new legislation*, CCH Editions.
UKCC (1987) *Confidentiality*.
UKCC (1992) *Code of Professional Conduct*, clauses 10, 13.

SUGGESTED READING CONCERNING CHILD ABUSE

Department of Health (1992) *Child Protection—Guidance for Senior Nurses, Health Visitors and Midwives*, HMSO, London.
HMSO (1991) *Working Together—Under the Children Act 1989*, Home Office *et al.*, HMSO, London.

There are numerous books and articles concerning child abuse. It is suggested that readers consult up-to-date literature, possibly starting with a selection from the reading list/references contained in the two documents above.

REFERENCES

Entries marked '*' are bibliographical entries rather than—or as well as—references.

*Beauchamp, T.L. and Childress, J.F. (1989) *Principles of Biomedical Ethics*, 3rd edn, Oxford University Press, Oxford, p.329.

*Benjamin, M. and Curtis, J. (1986) *Ethics in Nursing*, 2nd edn, Oxford University Press, Oxford.

*Brazier, M. (1987) *Medicine, Patients and the Law*, Penguin Books, Middlesex.

*Carlisle, D. (1991) To tell or not to tell. *Nursing Times*, **87**(16), 46–47.

*Carlisle, D. (1992) A clause for alarm? *Nursing Times*, **88**(24), 29–30.

*Department of Health (1992) *Child Protection—Guidance for Senior Nurses, Health Visitors and Midwives*, HMSO, London.

*Finch, J. (1989) Inside Law. *Nursing Standard*, **48**(3), 44–45.

*Freeman, M.D.A. (1988) *Medicine, Ethics and the Law*, Stevens and Sons, London.

*Gillon, R. (1986) *Philosophical Medical Ethics*, John Wiley and Sons, Chichester.

HMSO (1990) *Access to Health Records Act 1990*, HMSO, London.

*HMSO (1991) *Working Together—Under the Children Act 1989*, Home Office *et al.*, HMSO, London.

*Johnson, A.G. (1990) *Pathways in Medical Ethics*, Edward Arnold, London, p.76.

*Mason, J.K. and McCall Smith, R.A. (1987) *Law and Medical Ethics*, 2nd edn, Butterworths, London, pp.121, 164.

*Naish, J. (1989) In defence of whistleblowers. *Nursing Standard*, **49**(3), 21.

*Osborne, L.W. and Martin, C.M. (1989) The importance of listening to medical students' experiences when teaching them medical ethics. *Journal of Medical Ethics*, **15**, 35–38.

*Rowden, R. (1992) Self-imposed silence. *Nursing Times*, **88**(24), 26–29.

*Silverton, L. (1992) Confidence in cocaine. *MIDIRS Midwifery Digest*, **2**(2), 237–238.

*Sterling, J.L. (1984) *Data Protection Act 1984—A guide to the new legislation*, CCH Editions Ltd.

*Turner, T. (1992) The indomitable Mr Pink. *Nursing Times*, **88**(24), 26–29.

*UKCC (1987) *Confidentiality*.

*UKCC (1992) *Code of Professional Conduct*, clauses 10, 13.

3.

ACCOUNTABILITY

CASE STUDY

Ruth has been a community midwife for just over a year, having qualified two years prior to taking up this post. She recently conducted a booking interview in the home of one of her clients, according to policy. The couple lived in a two storey maisonette above a garage; as Ruth climbed the concrete steps, which were narrow and steep, she contemplated the difficulty facing this couple when manoeuvring a pram or pushchair.

Gillian was a 28-year-old primigravida of 11 weeks' gestation who was delighted about her pregnancy; her partner, Derek, was also present for the interview and he appeared to share Gillian's enthusiasm. During the interview Gillian indicated her intention to have a home confinement and Ruth asked her why she had made this decision. She discovered that Gillian had previously experienced a number of traumatic situations involving hospitals; she also felt that 'home' was the place where she wanted her baby to be born. When Derek was asked for his view, he stated that they had discussed the matter and he had decided to support Gillian's choice, despite the GP's refusal to accept her case.

Having determined Gillian's reasons, Ruth explained that, in this particular district, it was not considered suitable for a primigravida to have a home confinement. She gave a full explanation, while taking care not to frighten her, and, remembering her thoughts about the outside stairway, also explained that access to their home was not ideal if the emergency obstetric unit ('The Flying Squad') was required. She asked her to consider a DOMINO delivery, outlining what this entailed. Gillian was not deterred by this discussion but she did indicate that if a serious problem occurred during labour she would agree to be transferred to hospital. Derek stated that he understood Ruth's point of view but he felt he wanted to support Gillian in her decision, as she was the person most affected by the whole experience, especially as the hospital was only three miles away. Ruth explained that she would need to discuss the matter with her Supervisor of Midwives and she urged Gillian to find another general practitioner (GP) who would be prepared to accept her, explaining how she could do this.

When Ruth saw her Supervisor of Midwives, who was also the community manager, she explained the situation and requested that she be relieved of her duties to Gillian if she—Gillian—maintained her stance. Her reasons were that she did not consider Gillian to be suitable to deliver at home, particularly with poor access; also, she had never experienced a home confinement—not even as a student.

The Supervisor of Midwives said she would arrange to visit the couple, with Ruth, to discuss the matter further but that she would not relieve her of her duties to Gillian.

QUESTIONS FOR CONSIDERATION BY THE READER

1. Why did the Supervisor of Midwives need to visit the couple?

2. As an autonomous practitioner, did Ruth have the right to request relief from her duties in this case?

3. What was the probable reason for the Supervisor of Midwives' refusing the request?

4. What would Ruth's responsibilities be in preparation for this confinement?

5. If a complication were to occur during labour, resulting in morbidity or mortality of mother or baby, could Ruth be held accountable for it?

An issue that is not discussed here, but which readers may wish to pursue, is choice of place of confinement.

Question 1. Why did the Supervisor of Midwives need to visit the couple?

Two specific aspects of the role of the Supervisor of Midwives are to protect the interests of the public and to support the midwives for whom she provides supervision. In this case the interests of the woman and the midwife seem to be in conflict. In order to support both sides, the Supervisor of Midwives must visit the couple, if they will allow this, preferably with the midwife concerned. She needs to listen to the woman's point of view and determine that she has made an informed decision. In order to do this she should reinforce the procedure that the midwife would have undertaken. This would include giving all the possibilities for confinement, outlining the advantages and disadvantages of each, and giving the results of any recent research into the place of confinement. She would also need to explain how Gillian's obstetric status could affect these options (ASM, 1989). Assuming that Gillian's decision was unchanged and that she exhibited full understanding of what she was undertaking, the Supervisor of Midwives would have no choice but to agree to provide adequate midwifery cover. She would then complete her own records of the situation; this would include writing to the couple to confirm her understanding of what took place in the interview and the decisions that were made.

It could be said that not a lot is achieved in such a visit, that all the Supervisor of Midwives has done is assess whether the midwife has carried out her initial duties correctly, followed by giving the couple a 'stamp of approval'. On the contrary, a lot has been achieved. She has shown the couple that she is supporting them in their decision, having already given her views on the safety of the situation—she is therefore fulfilling her duty to the public. In reinforcing what the midwife had previously discussed with the couple, she is indicating her support for her as well; she will also have assessed the situation that is facing the midwife so that she can offer relevant support. It is probably true that she has also assessed the midwife's handling of the situation; not only is it her duty to do so, in order to protect the public, but she is then in a position to support fully the midwife's actions if any problems occur or complaints are made.

Question 2. As an autonomous practitioner, did Ruth have the right to request relief from her duties in this case?

Although many readers may sympathize with Ruth in this situation, she did not have the right to refuse to care for this woman, which is what her request was seeking to authorize. As a midwife she:

> ... must be able to give the necessary supervision, care and advice to women during pregnancy, labour and the postpartum period, to conduct deliveries on (his) own responsibility ...

> (UKCC, 1991a)

Also, she is:

> ... accountable for (his) own practice in whatever environment (he) practises.

Although 99% of deliveries take place in hospital, any midwife accepting a community post must be aware that they might be required to attend a home confinement, planned or otherwise. In taking up this post then, Ruth was accepting the complete responsibilities attendant on such a post.

It could be said that Ruth was adhering to rule 40(2) of the *Midwives Rules* (UKCC, 1991b) and the *Code of Professional Conduct* (UKCC, 1992a) in that she is not prepared to undertake something for which she feels inadequately trained. To a point this is commendable but it needs to be determined exactly what it is that she has not been trained for. It appears to be the confinement itself that she is concerned about. This entails monitoring the condition of mother and fetus and the progress of labour, also delivery of the fetus by the use of skilled technique, delivery of the placenta and membranes with control of haemorrhage (by active or passive means) followed by observation and continued care of the mother. It also involves assessment of the neonate, with any necessary resuscitative measures, plus observation and continued care. Any complications that arise should be notified to a medical practitioner.

Attention to the administration of drugs, and record-keeping, are also important aspects to be included. Everything mentioned here is included in the theory and practice of all midwifery education and training programmes, including the theory—and practice for some—relating to home confinement; therefore there is nothing for which Ruth can say she is inadequately trained. It is mainly a matter of her applying all the principles to a different setting.

Question 3. What was the probable reason for the Supervisor of Midwives' refusing the request?

The most probable reason for the Supervisor of Midwives to refuse Ruth's request was the knowledge that she owed a duty of care to her client and she had no 'reasonable justification' for relinquishing that duty (Dimond, 1989). She may also have considered Ruth's development and decided that this was an ideal opportunity for her to gain the experience that was lacking.

Question 4. What would Ruth's responsibilities be in preparation for this confinement?

Ruth will be accountable for her practice; it is therefore her responsibility for providing the safest care possible within the limits of what is available to her. Firstly, she will need to update herself on how to conduct a home delivery. Apart from making use of her nearest midwifery library and a link tutor if there is one, she should read the local policies regarding the management of such a confinement, discussing any areas of concern with her Supervisor of Midwives (UKCC, 1991a; 1992b). There is plenty of time before Gillian's estimated date of delivery, therefore, if it has been a long time since Ruth last attended a woman in labour, she could request—or the Supervisor of Midwives could suggest—that she conducts at least one case in the local maternity unit (ASM, 1989). This would preferably be a 'low-risk' case where traditional tactile skills alone could be employed (hands, eyes and ears, with the aid of a Pinard's stethoscope). Another possibility would be to arrange to attend a home confinement with another midwife even if this meant communication with the Supervisor of Midwives and midwives of a neighbouring authority.

In some authorities it is policy that a second midwife is called at the approach of the second stage of labour. Whether or not this is the policy in this particular authority, the Supervisor of Midwives is required to adopt this approach in this particular case, in order to provide support and assistance (Cronk and Flint, 1990; ASM, 1989).

Apart from conducting routine antenatal care and education, Ruth will be responsible for preparing Gillian for her confinement at home. This will include possible recommendations regarding the positioning of furniture, protection of the bed and floor, and provision of any equipment (a bowl, a bucket, towels, etc.) as well as the obvious baby items. Access to hot and cold running water and a telephone, plus some method of heating the room, would be desirable. One might normally say these were essential, but as the woman will be staying at home anyway, dictating that these are essentials seems pointless. The couple can be reassured that the provision of gallons of hot water will not be necessary—other than for hygiene purposes and making tea or coffee. Ruth will need to know whether Gillian has managed to secure the services of a GP. If she has failed to do this then Ruth or the Supervisor of Midwives could try to do so. When the time comes, if there is no GP cover, then Ruth would contact a local on-call GP and/or the emergency obstetric unit, if required. The Department of Health's *The Health Committee Second Report on the Maternity Services* (1992) makes a number of recommendations with regard to GPs and intra-partum care, one such recommendation being that GP cover should be arranged if a woman in that practice desires it (para. 349).

Question 5. If a complication were to occur during labour, resulting in morbidity or mortality of mother or baby, could Ruth be held accountable for it?

Ruth can only be held responsible for her own actions and omissions; she cannot be held accountable for complications that are beyond her control. For instance, if fetal distress occurs despite normal progress in labour and adequate care and observation by Ruth, then she is not at fault. If, however, fetal distress occurs because Ruth has failed to diagnose 'failure to progress', or has noticed it but has not sought medical aid, then she is accountable for this omission. The same would be true regarding post-partum haemorrhage (PPH): if active or passive management is carried out properly but still a PPH occurs, then she is not at fault; however, mismanagement of the third stage of labour, resulting in a PPH, could be attributable to her. If the complication results in morbidity or mortality of either mother or baby, then Ruth will again be judged by her actions (or lack of them); if she has followed accepted procedures and summoned medical aid then she has not been negligent. Gillian has agreed to be transferred to hospital if a serious problem arises (one could speculate as to what she would consider 'serious'…) but when the time comes she could refuse to allow Ruth to call a doctor. If this occurs, then again, if Ruth follows the accepted procedures, documenting everything as fully as she can and reporting to the Supervisor of Midwives as soon as possible, she cannot be held responsible for a poor outcome. In the event that a doctor attends the confinement, by choice or request, then Ruth will still be accountable for any action or omission of hers, even if following the doctor's instructions. Accountability cannot be transferred. By carrying out the instruction, Ruth would, in effect, be agreeing with it and therefore would be accountable for it.

Further Discussion

If a group of students or qualified midwives is asked for a definition of accountability, in the author's experience it is usual to hear 'responsibility for one's actions', which of course is quite right. It is possible, however, that the importance of this still does not fully 'sink in'. In Oxford dictionaries, of various types and dates, it equates to 'responsibility', however, Roget's *Thesaurus* (1980) creates a deeper perspective:

Liability	*Duty*
lay oneself open to...	moral obligation
stand a chance of ...	onus
at the mercy of ...	conscientiousness
responsible	answerable
	responsible

'Responsibility' is the common factor, but one would do well to remember the other terms used.

For *whom and what is the midwife accountable?*

It is obvious that the women and their foetuses/babies feature high on the list, with midwives being responsible for their safety and general well-being, including educating the women in safe care of their babies. There is also responsibility for the family as a whole; midwives are ideally placed to tackle aspects of health promotion with or for the whole family. It is also their duty to observe for, and assist with, the healthy integration of the baby into the family, thus helping to prevent some of the physical and mental traumas that can occur, particularly for the mother and baby, if integration is delayed.

In some respects all midwives are accountable for their colleagues, of all grades, in maintaining safe and harmonious teamwork. Observance of general 'health and safety' principles are essential, such as giving proper attention to the disposal of sharp objects and care when dealing with body fluids. As for harmony, if this is lacking then it can create a stressful working atmosphere, which not only may affect the health and well-being of the staff but could affect the care received by the clients and certainly would create a bad image to clients and their visitors.

The 'what' in the question generally relates to equipment. Technological equipment is expensive and often temperamental through over-use; it should be handled with care. It should be remembered that the appropriate technicians are the only people who are approved to correct the faults (many of which could be prevented by responsible handling) not a midwife who is handy with a screwdriver or a blade from her scissors! Machinery is often used and abused by many, even the husbands at times, therefore the midwife can only be held responsible for any specific damage or negligence caused by her.

The above points are slightly different from actual accountability; however, the midwife *is* accountable for any acts and omissions pertaining to these areas—it therefore seems logical to include them here.

Accountability is one of the areas that is highlighted in discussions regarding the difference between midwifery and nursing. In looking through the above areas of responsibility, the reader could be forgiven for considering that there is no difference in accountability; in fact the next three areas are those that create the difference.

Under the *Congenital Disabilities (Civil Liability) Act 1976* (HMSO, 1976), a midwife can be held accountable for any act or omission committed by her that has resulted in damage to the fetus or baby. Action can be taken on behalf of the child, up to the age of 18. Once the child reaches 18, action must be taken by that person up to the age of 21. If the person, once adult, is considered mentally incompetent, then an advocate can act as a representative. It can take up to four years for the case to reach the courts, therefore a midwife could be in the position of having to interpret her records up to 25 years after the event. This in itself indicates the need for full and accurate record keeping. The effects of this Act were expected to relate to cases occurring after the Act came into force, however, the Court of Appeal has recently ruled that two cases, where injury occurred prior to the Act, can continue with their claim under common law (Dyer, 1992).

Midwives are permitted to carry and prescribe certain drugs. Their exemption from the *Misuse of Drugs Act 1971* (HMSO, 1971) permits them to carry out specific functions with particular drugs. This must only be in accordance with their sphere of practice—they cannot, for instance, give intramuscular pethidine to a client's husband who is in severe pain from renal colic. Although there is the facility for midwives to carry various drugs, they do not necessarily do so. They must abide by local policies regarding the actual drugs and quantities that they carry.

There is also specific accountability with regard to notification and registration of births and deaths. It is usually the midwife who notifies the birth that she has attended, within 36 hours, and the mother and/or father who register(s) the baby within 42 days of the birth. If the parents neglect to register the baby, then it is the duty of the midwife. This does not mean that she needs to seek them out at 41 days after delivery, rather she would be contacted by the Registrar's office. The personnel in this office would know to await the registration, as the birth had already been notified. As for deaths, it would normally be the responsibility of the doctor who certified the mother, viable fetus or neonate dead who would complete the death or stillbirth certificate and issue it to the family for them to register the death. If a registered medical practitioner is not available for some reason, then the duty falls to the midwife present at the delivery; so too does the duty to register the death if the family fail to do so (UKCC, 1991a).

These points are obviously extra to the 16 contained in the *Code of Professional Conduct* (UKCC, 1992a).

To *whom is the midwife accountable?*

Firstly she is accountable to the family, of which the mother is an integral member. A breach in her duties to mother or baby resulting in either of them suffering harm could cause them to sue her in the civil courts.

She is accountable to the UKCC for her conduct and it is for the Professional Conduct Committee of the council to determine whether the midwife is guilty of conduct unworthy of a midwife, and therefore guilty of misconduct (Dimond, 1989); such a verdict could result in the midwife being removed from the register (UKCC, 1990). The investigation and disciplinary process begins with the Supervisor of Midwives. The UKCC produced an advisory document in 1989—*Exercising Accountability*—which seeks to assist practitioners in this important area. Accountability to her employer is the next consideration. A midwife is contracted to carry out the duties for which she is employed in accordance with the statutory rules and codes; also, she must adhere to the local policies within the employing authority. Any breach of duty to the woman and/or baby in her care could be considered to be a breach in contract, thus resulting in possible dismissal.

The last, but very important, person to be considered is the midwife herself. The author firmly believes that accountability to oneself should not be dismissed as unimportant in the face of other agents of accountability. Everyone makes mistakes, some more regrettable than others, but whether or not these mistakes are 'punished' by another agency, the knowledge of that error will stay with that midwife forever, a fact she should keep in mind throughout her professional activities.

As this century has progressed, the face of midwifery has changed. Although the principles behind accountability are largely the same, the variety of activities in which a midwife may be involved has blossomed. Not all midwives are involved in all the new aspects but they are obviously accountable for their part in any that they undertake. These activities include provision of contraceptive advice, preconception counselling, ultrasound scanning, perineal suturing, epidural 'top-ups', venepuncture and, in some cases, siting venflons/IVIs. With the advent of electronic fetal monitoring, midwives have had to learn how to use the machinery and interpret the readings. Midwives now deliver most women in hospital, often at a time dictated by the doctors, at the same time as trying to observe the autonomy of these women.

One of the most difficult areas faced by midwives is probably the observance of clause 2.2.10 in A *Midwife's Code of Practice* (1991a) which states:

> ... *to carry out treatment prescribed by a doctor.*

This is particularly difficult when that doctor may only just be starting in obstetric experience. Obviously midwives are at liberty to discuss decisions made by such doctors and can often offer advice but much depends on the doctor's willingness to accept the advice and the midwife's manner in giving it. In some units, it would appear, junior doctors are considered 'junior' to the experienced midwives; in others, such doctors are not permitted to make decisions in the delivery suite—unless of a general medical nature. The author would suggest that midwives should not find the above clause so difficult to put in to practice. There are many situations where the 'treatments prescribed' are concerned with 'high-risk' cases or non-midwifery/obstetric matters, where it is the doctor's province anyway. In the midwifery/obstetric field, if the midwife feels that she cannot carry out the doctor's wishes then she should not do so. She should explain why she feels unable to do so, for instance 'I cannot rupture the membranes, as to do so with a high presenting part is dangerous', inviting the doctor to either change the instruction or conduct the procedure personally. It is worth repeating that accountability cannot be transferred; if the midwife did rupture the membranes and a cord prolapse occurred, resulting in a stillbirth, it would be useless for her to stand up in court and state 'The doctor told me to.' The doctor may well be guilty of an error of judgement but an error no greater than the midwife who carried out what she knew to be an unsafe procedure (UKCC, 1992a, b).

APPLYING THE THEORIES

A utilitarian view

The client is choosing to have a home confinement with or without Ruth. The outcome of this, therefore, does not feature in the decision. If Ruth was allowed to relinquish her responsibility then the client would need to begin to relate to another midwife; the first midwife would be initially relieved at the lifting of the responsibility but she would still be lacking in important experience.

If she fulfils her responsibilities then the client will maintain the same carer with whom she booked, without involving another midwife unnecessarily. The midwife concerned will have been updated and will get the experience that she needs. The balance is slightly in favour of continuing with the case.

A deontological view

The midwife has a duty to care for this woman, which also includes updating herself. The decision would be to continue.

SUGGESTED READING

Dimond, B. (1989) Accountability in the legal context. *Nursing Standard,* **3**(49).

Heywood Jones, I. (1989) Stretched to the limits. *Nursing Times,* **85**(46), 38–39.

Jenkins, R. and Murphy, A. (1991) *Accountability, the Law and the Midwife,* DLC, South Bank University, London.

Kargar, I. (1990) Traditional midwifery skills *Nursing Times*, **86**(23), 74–75.

Rumbold, R. (1991) *Ethics in Nursing and Midwifery Practice*, DLC, South Bank University, London.

UKCC (1989) *Exercising Accountability*.

UKCC (1990) '... *with a view to removal from the register?...*'

UKCC (1991a) *A Midwife's Code of Practice*.

UKCC (1991b) *Midwives Rules*.

UKCC (1992a) *Code of Professional Conduct*.

UKCC (1992b) *The Scope of Professional Practice*.

REFERENCES

Entries marked '*' are bibliographical entries rather than—or as well as—references.

*ASM (1989) *Supervision of Midwives—The whys and wherefores*.

*Chamberlain, G. and Orr, C. (eds)(1990) *How To Avoid Medico-legal Problems in Obstetrics and Gynaecology*, The Chameleon Press, London.

*Cole, A. (1991) Upholding the code. *Nursing Times*, **87**(27), 26–29.

*Cronk, M. and Flint, C. (1990) *Community Midwifery*, Butterworth Heinemann Ltd, Oxford.

*Dimond, B. (1989) Accountability in the legal context. *Nursing Standard*, **3**(49), 29–30.

Department of Health (1992) *The Health Committee Second Report on the Maternity Services*, para. 349, HMSO, London.

Dyer, C. (1992) New ruling may fuel surge in birth damage cases. *BMJ*, **304**(6832), 937.

*Heywood Jones, I. (1989) Stretched to the limits. *Nursing Times*, **85**(46), 38–39.

HMSO (1971) *Misuse of Drugs Act 1971*, HMSO, London.

HMSO (1976) *Congenital Disabilities (Civil Liability) Act 1976*, HMSO, London.

*Isherwood, K. (1988) Friend or watchdog? *Nursing Times*, **84**(24), 65.

*Jenkins, R. and Murphy, A. (1991) *Accountability, the Law and the Midwife*, DLC, South Bank University, London.

*Kargar, I. (1990) Traditional midwifery skills *Nursing Times*, **86**(23), 74–75.

*Lansdell, M. (1989) Friend and counsellor. *Nursing Times*, **85**(28), 76.

*NHS, *The named midwife*, The Patient's Charter Group.

Roget, P.M. (1980) Roget's Thesaurus of Synonyms and Antonyms, College Books, London.

*Rumbold, R. (1991) *Ethics in Nursing and Midwifery Practice*, DLC, South Bank University, London.

*UKCC (1989) *Exercising Accountability*.

*UKCC (1990) '... *with a view to removal from the register?...*'

*UKCC (1991a) *A Midwife's Code of Practice*.

*UKCC (1991b) *Midwives Rules*.

*UKCC (1992a) *Code of Professional Conduct*.

*UKCC (1992b) *The Scope of Professional Practice*.

4.

AUTONOMY AND CONSENT

CASE STUDY

Denise is 22 years old and has just experienced childbirth for the first time. Her pregnancy was uneventful, other than the early ultrasound scan report stating that the baby was due two weeks earlier than Denise expected. She and her husband David attended the various classes for Preparation for Parenthood and were very interested in the idea of preparing a 'birthplan'. This had been discussed at one of the classes and the midwife was prepared to assist couples in this preparation. They explained to her that they wanted labour to be 'normal', without interventions if at all possible, but they did not want to antagonize anybody as they were aware that the professionals knew best. They had included that they would be willing to consider any action required if the need arose—they just wanted to be involved in the decision-making process.

At 40 weeks plus two days, Denise started labour spontaneously. On arrival at the hospital all observations were normal, her cervix was dilated 4 cm and she was coping well with her contractions. The midwife caring for Denise read the birthplan and stated that she would do her best to comply with their wishes. She indicated that the policy in that unit was to artificially rupture the membranes when labour was established (at 3–4 cm). At Denise's request she explained the reasons for this:

- To observe the 'water' (liquor) in case the baby should become distressed.
- To be able to monitor the baby's heart rate directly, instead of through the abdomen.
- To speed up the labour.

The external tracing of the baby's heart rate was very clear and Denise was content to be monitored if she could also move around; it was decided, therefore, that artificial rupture of the membranes should not be performed at this stage.

After three hours, the obstetric Senior House Officer (SHO) on duty came to assess her progress, according to unit policy. On checking the labour notes he noted that the membranes were still intact; he challenged the midwife regarding failure to follow policy and she advised him of the woman's wishes. On examination, the doctor found the cervix to be dilated 6 cm, he asked for an amnihook; the midwife was hesitant but the doctor was quietly insistent. Denise became aware of the tension in the room and, on asking what was wrong, the midwife replied 'Nothing, baby seems fine!'; the doctor carried out the procedure. The husband asked what the doctor was doing but it was too late.

Labour progressed normally although it now became more painful and Denise required pain relief which she had been managing to avoid. After another three hours, a normal female baby was delivered and both mother and baby recovered well.

Denise and David complained in writing that:

- Their wishes had not been considered by the doctor.
- Unnecessary intervention had been undertaken without their consent, particularly Denise's.
- They felt deceived by their midwife, although they accepted that she was acting under the doctor's instruction and she had provided good care.

QUESTIONS FOR CONSIDERATION BY THE READER

1. Was the doctor at liberty to disregard the couple's views?

2. Could the midwife have prevented the situation from arising?

3. Whether or not she could have prevented the situation, could she have prevented the couple from feeling deceived by her?

4. Are their complaints well founded; is there a case to answer?

Issues that are not discussed here, but which readers may wish to pursue, are privacy, the uninvited involvement of doctors in low-risk cases, and assertiveness. Truth-telling and advocacy could be looked at in more depth.

Question 1. Was the doctor at liberty to disregard the couple's views?

To answer this question, it is necessary to determine the status of the couple: could they be considered to be autonomous? It would appear that they had been a motivated couple in the antenatal period. They had attended Preparation for Parenthood classes and become interested in the concept of a birthplan. They had sought professional advice from the midwife in order to formulate their plan. Although they preferred not to have interventions, they stated that their main request was that they be involved in any decision making.

This would appear to confirm their autonomy as a couple, as they exhibited rational, self-governed and self-controlled behaviour. They also requested and received, from the midwife in attendance at the labour, information relating to the reasons for artificially rupturing the fetal membranes. They did not, however, receive information regarding the benefits of their remaining intact. It is generally accepted that intact membranes create a barrier against intra-uterine infection and assist in the dilatation of the cervix; it is also known to prevent prolapse of the umbilical cord in cases where the fetal presentation is 'poorly fitting'. As rupture of the membranes causes an increase in the production of prostaglandins, which in turn creates greater contraction of the myometrium, labour is often considered to be more painful following this occurrence. Therefore, in a labour that is progressing normally, it would seem to cause an unnecessary increase in pain. A number of commentators have also highlighted the following advantages (among others): maintenance of hydrostatic pressure in the uterus and protection of the umbilical cord from compression, and therefore prevention of fetal distress (Gabbe *et al.*, 1976; Dunn, 1978; Smythe, 1974).

The doctor cannot consider the 'couple' in this situation—he has a duty of care to his patient, in this case Denise. The fetus is not considered a patient (see 'Maternal versus fetal rights'). It is therefore Denise's autonomy that must be confirmed and it is necessary to consider the conditions under which she would possibly be considered to have a temporary loss of autonomy, i.e. when she might be considered irrational in her thought or behaviour. As there is no indication that Denise has a psychiatric condition, the most likely situation for appearing irrational would be following narcotic injection (for pain relief in labour), which she did not require prior to the doctor's intervention. Another possibility would be the suspicion that Denise was acting under pressure from David, thus disputing the autonomy of her requests. This occasionally happens and it is very difficult to deal with—there would appear to be no such indication in this situation. Sometimes women have misguided ideas of what is 'natural' and therefore right, but this situation does not occur here either.

The Handbook of Medical Ethics (BMA, 1986) states:

> *Doctors offer advice but it is the patient who decides whether or not to accept the advice.*

It is accepted that doctors have autonomy of practice, making their own decisions regarding their choice of management of cases, but the previous statement, added to the confirmation of Denise's autonomy, would indicate that the doctor was not at liberty to disregard the stated views. Having done so he has acted paternalistically, therefore denying the woman's autonomy.

Within his duty of care lies the doctor's duty to help his patient: beneficence. There is also a stronger duty—in most cases—to do no harm: nonmaleficence (Faulder, 1985). It could be argued that the doctor obeyed neither of these principles in this situation as, following his intervention, her labour became more painful and she required pain relief. It would be impossible to assess whether or not Denise would have eventually needed the pain relief but it is commonly accepted by practitioners that contractions become more painful following rupture of the membranes (Flint, 1990; NCT, 1989; Henderson, 1990).

The first principle considered here was that of autonomy. The next principle is that of informed consent, i.e. whether Denise was given sufficient information on which to base her decision. (Both principles are explained in 'Further discussion'.) The midwife gave Denise all the basic reasons for performing artificial rupture of the membranes. She even indicated the unit's policy, although it did not feature as an individual reason, more as an 'umbrella' for the list that followed. It could be said, therefore, that Denise had made an informed refusal to the procedure—following the examination and consultation with her midwife—on admission. It was stated in the birthplan that Denise would be willing to consider any action required, if it became necessary; but the need had not arisen by the time the doctor arrived. It would appear that he attended as a matter of routine, not because he was summoned by the midwife, therefore there was no problem perceived by her. In fact, the doctor based his initial judgement regarding the membranes on the labour notes, challenging the midwife on failure to follow policy, also, therefore, failing to recognize the midwife's autonomy of practice. It was at this stage that he was made aware of Denise's wishes and initial refusal—he was therefore aware that her consent was being withheld before he examined her.

In this case there appears to have been no problem with regard to what is usually considered necessary practice during labour. Denise, unlike some women, probably accepted that there was implied consent for certain examinations (Dimond, 1990). This would mean that she accepted these examinations as part of having her baby, whereas actual interventions she did not. Perhaps the doctor judged that Denise would probably give subsequent consent. Carter (1977) lists a number of considerations that would be central to making this judgement; she then states:

> It is highly unlikely that anyone will subsequently consent to a paternalistic act which will not harmonize with his permanent aims and preferences. And if the act were contrary to the subject's known preferences he would rightly see the interference as an outright assault on the integrity of his person.

There is nothing to suggest that the doctor or midwife had found anything abnormal in the well-being of either mother or fetus; in fact the examination revealed good progress. This would suggest that the only reason for the doctor to perform the artificial rupture of the membranes was unit policy. Regardless of the reason, the fact is he did not make any attempt to elicit Denise's wishes at that time; it is possible, though unlikely, that she may have been willing to give consent to artificial rupture of the membranes—if he had given good reason for it. It would appear that the doctor chose to ignore the need for his patient's consent to such an intervention. Gillett (1989) suggests that, in scrutinizing the actions of this doctor, we ask:

> i) whether he appreciated the moral demand;
> ii) whether he acted with an endorsable set of values; and
> iii) whether he acted sincerely.

Readers might care to determine the answer to these questions. It would be necessary to identify the 'moral demand' of the situation; presumably this would include the moral obligation to respect Denise's autonomy and gain informed consent before performing any procedures, especially one for which she has already withheld her consent. If it is thought that the doctor acted in accordance with (ii) then this is approving the practice of paternalism and allowing an assault to be made; in fact it is possible that a charge of battery could be made (a civil suit), not for the examination but for the actual rupturing of membranes without consent (Mason and McCall Smith, 1987). The final point deals with his sincerity; it is possible to accept that he acted sincerely, in his adherence to the unit's policy, but his sincerity to the code of medical ethics, laid down by the BMA, is less clear.

Artificial rupture of the membranes is a contentious issue and, while the debate will not be entered into here, it is worth noting that most midwives and doctors who profess to be against routine performance of the procedure give clinical rather than ethical reasons.

It would, perhaps, be helpful to reconsider the reasons for amniotomy to be performed. The midwife explained the reasons as:

• To observe the 'water' (liquor) in case the baby should become distressed.
• To be able to monitor the baby's heart rate directly, instead of through the abdomen.
• To speed up the labour.

A Canadian study—September 1987 to September 1988—failed to support this assumption (Fraser *et al.*, 1991). The survey was of 3000 mothers who delivered in 1987 and, although the methodology was dubious (which they admit) they suggest that their findings indicate that aspects of labour management with regard to artificial rupture of the membranes need review.

This is a fair summary of reasons in this particular case (as induction of labour would not have been required for Denise) but researchers have highlighted the use of another reason. The National Childbirth Trust (NCT) conducted a survey in 1989—by self-completion questionnaire— because of the experiences of women which were reported by an NCT teacher in Putney and Fulham.

This survey showed that the actual incidence of artificial rupture of the membranes was unknown because hospital records were inconsistent regarding the procedure. They also discovered that the reasons given were as mentioned above, but 'as routine' also featured. The study by Robinson *et al.* (1983) highlighted the fact that unit policy was the greatest dictator with regard to artificial rupture of the membranes, followed closely by the midwife's decision.

It could be argued, however, that many midwives will follow unit policy without questioning its wisdom, as a matter of routine; if this is so, then the figures obtained for unit policy should be even higher. Henderson (1990) found this to be the case in her small study in 1984 involving observation of labours followed by interviews of the mothers and midwives. She states in her findings that there was:

A misconception on the part of the midwives that they were using their own judgement while in fact they were unwittingly following a routine in part due to medical pressure.

Question 2. Could the midwife have prevented the situation from arising?

The midwife's role in this case needs to be examined. Midwives are encouraged to consider their role to be multi-facetted; terms such as practitioner (or care-giver), counsellor, friend, advisor, educator and advocate are commonly used in order that areas of care and responsibility are not omitted. It would appear that it was the roles of advocate and friend that were lacking in this situation. Midwives often fear the consequences of 'disobeying' a doctor or questioning that doctor's orders or actions, but their accountability to the women in their care, themselves and their professional body, requires that they do this when the need arises. In the Royal College of Midwives Trust (RCM) document *Practical Guidance for Midwives Facing Ethical or Moral Dilemmas* it states:

> *The midwife is involved in treatment prescribed by doctors which she has the right to question if she considers this to be contrary to the interests of mother and baby, or in contravention of the law. It must be emphasised that working within a team structure does not absolve the midwife from her individual responsibility and accountability.*

They are required to be professional at all times and this creates another problem: much of what is decided—particularly in labour—for the woman occurs at the bedside. Questioning the doctor in the view or hearing of the woman, and her birth companion, could mean the loss of confidence in either or both professionals. Generally, this could be prevented by adequate discussion, involving all relevant parties, and joint decision making. This would entail giving full information, leading to informed consent or refusal, assuming that the professionals would remember to act on it. This could also indicate the need for doctors and midwives to discuss hypothetical cases; this would produce a professional airing of differences and suitable agreement of policies and procedures, thus preventing many of the conflicts.

As the woman's advocate, it was the midwife's duty to make it clear to the doctor, in the woman's hearing, that consent to artificial rupture of the membranes had not been given. Once he asked for the required instrument with which to perform the procedure, she should have refused, reminding him of Denise's wishes and suggesting he discuss the matter with Denise. As a 'friend', the midwife should have considered Denise's feelings; instead, she acted against her by 'aiding and abetting' in a morally wrong act. The midwife, as an accountable professional, cannot pass on accountability to others. Although it was the doctor who actually performed the procedure, the midwife was aware that he was acting against the woman's wishes and she could at least have objected more strongly.

Question 3. Whether or not she could have prevented the situation, could she have prevented the couple from feeling deceived by her?

It is difficult to determine whether or not the midwife could have prevented the couple from feeling deceived by her. The fact is she did deceive them—not only did she not openly object to the actions of the doctor but she lied when questioned by Denise as to what the doctor was doing. Immoral behaviour is not only achieved by our actions but by our omissions to act. This 'acts and omissions' doctrine is accepted in law, with court recognition that:

> ... a crime can be committed by omission if a duty to act is present.
>
> (Beauchamp and Childress, 1989)

The midwife initially acted correctly in pointing out Denise's views to the doctor, unfortunately she was then guilty of an act and an omission against the interests of the woman for whose care she was responsible. Her duty to act was clear but she failed to do so, she then compounded this by participating in the procedure, by handing the equipment to the doctor and evading the issue when asked what was wrong.

The midwife abdicated her responsibility to the couple in favour of the demands of the doctor. The only way in which she could have prevented this was to indicate to the couple what the doctor's intention was, thus giving them the opportunity to refuse. Had this occurred, the actual incident would probably have been avoided.

Question 4. Are their complaints well founded; is there a case to answer?

With regard to the complaints made by Denise and David, it is necessary to consider whether there is a case to answer. The first point is obviously true: the doctor did not show any indication of considering their views. Gillon (1986) in summarizing his passage on the doctor–patient relationship states:

> ... the principle of respect for autonomy asks the doctor to have at the back of his mind the question, Would the patient ... wish me to do what I am doing or intend to do? If not, How can I justify doing it? Usually the best way to answer the first question is to ask the person concerned.

For the second point, we know that he carried out the intervention, but was it 'unnecessary'? On the basis of the indicators previously mentioned, there was evidence to suggest that progress was normal, therefore no intervention was required for acceleration. It would appear that the fetal heart rate was recording well via the abdominal route as there was no indication of internal monitoring occurring after artificial rupture of the membranes. As there was no sign of fetal distress, there was no indication to observe the colour of the liquor. This would suggest that the intervention was only necessary from the point of following unit policy, surely no real indication. The WHO report *Appropriate Technology for Birth* (1985) includes 15 recommendations; it is interesting that number five states:

> *Artificial early rupture of the membranes, as a routine process, is not scientifically justified.*

It has already been ascertained that the artificial rupture of the membranes was performed without consent. This, in civil law, would be deemed battery and it would appear unlikely that a satisfactory defence could be made (Brazier, 1987).

The last point in the letter of complaint relates to the deception by the midwife. The relationship between a labouring woman and her midwife is thought, by most of those concerned, to be very special. It is a relationship based on trust—the woman entrusts herself and her (as yet unborn) baby into the care of a professional who should be able to guide her through an often arduous event. For some women this 'guiding' is as paternalistic as it sounds, as they have made the autonomous decision to hand over the majority of the decision making to the person who they feel knows best. In other cases, as with Denise, women have carefully selected the path they wish to follow during this major life experience, and they are looking to the midwife to assist them in the safe achievement of their plans. It should also be stated here that trust should be two-way; the woman had made an informed, autonomous decision and the midwife should trust the mother to continue to make such decisions as the need arises. The midwife in this case started her care of Denise well; she indicated her intention to follow the birthplan and, in doing this, she was creating the basis for the correct partnership in labour care. She will have given Denise a feeling of security, thus encouraging her to relax into her labour.

Half-way through the labour, however, there was a sudden change in the atmosphere of this partnership with the arrival of the doctor. The midwife became defensive of her own actions, having been challenged about the intact membranes. She then broke her agreement with Denise by not 'doing her best to comply with their wishes'. She could have acted on their behalf, all she needed to do was inform Denise of what was about to happen, giving her the chance to question the doctor and then make her own decision. What she should have done was challenge the doctor and refuse to take part in the procedure, giving a proper explanation of her actions. She could also have summoned a more senior midwife (if there was one), the Registrar on duty, or her Supervisor of Midwives, and obviously she would need to document the incident appropriately. As a qualified midwife she should not follow any instructions from a doctor if she feels that it is inappropriate—as it was in this case— nor should she fail to respect the woman's autonomy by lying to her (UKCC, 1989).

There can be no doubt that, for whatever reason, she deceived them. Thankfully she gave good care apart from that, so there was a positive aspect to Denise's labour—other than her baby.

Faulder (1985), in her book *Whose Body Is It?*, states:

> *Giving our informed consent to medical treatment is the ultimate expression of the responsibility each one of us has for our own person ... Our bodies belong to us. They are who we are.*

The author suggests that it will take a long time for all health professionals to come to terms with informed consent, and much longer still where informed refusal is concerned! (There are at least two other points for the reader to consider in this case, although they will not be considered any further here: privacy, and why there should be a policy for SHOs to oversee all women in the delivery suite.)

FURTHER DISCUSSION

Autonomy

Downie and Calman (1987) define autonomy as:

> *To be an autonomous person is to have the ability to be able to formulate and carry out one's own plans or policies. [...] A second feature ... is the ability to govern one's conduct by rules or values.*

Some traits of this principle may be familiar to parents of adolescents as they are usually involved in encouraging their offspring to 'stand on their own feet', 'know what they want', 'make up their own minds' and 'have an aim in life' (Downie and Calman, 1987).

To be autonomous, then, means being in control of one's life—self-governing and self-ruled. This includes behaving rationally (in Kant's view this is the essence of personhood) and being in control of one's liberty and freedom. Autonomy and freedom are not the same; under the heading of freedom we could say 'Let them do what they want to', while under autonomy we would say 'Let them act freely, but they should be able to give reasons for their actions.' The following example puts this into a more practical setting:

A man requests a rabies injection—which is extremely painful and unpleasant, and possibly expensive too! When the doctor asked him why, the man replied '... because it seems a good idea'.

This does not appear to be a rational reason, therefore the injection would probably not be given. If, in the same situation, the man was to reply '... because yesterday I was bitten by a dog, in Spain.' (Walker, 1990; pers. comm.) it would be a rational reason and the injection would almost certainly be advised.

It is important to consider whether autonomy is a principle that we would wish to uphold. Deontologists may well consider that there can be no negotiation regarding autonomy, it is an intrinsic value of deontology and therefore always a priority. This follows Kant's view that people are ends in themselves and should not be regarded merely as a means to someone else's ends (Benjamin and Curtis, 1986). With this in mind, it is important to consider the woman's goals not the practitioner's. In the given situation, it would be reasonable to assume that the woman's goal was to achieve a successful outcome to her labour, without any intervention and undue haste. The practitioner's goal could have been to get the woman delivered of her baby before the shift ended—almost as a reward for that practitioner's efforts. It could also be envisaged that the quicker the labour, the quicker the list of women awaiting induction could be reduced. Such goals would create incompatibility between the woman and the practitioner. Failure to act in accordance with the woman's goal, without her informed consent, would be a rejection of her autonomy (Beauchamp and Childress, 1989).

Utilitarians, on the other hand, would examine the benefits that might be promoted by it, not only to the woman but to the practitioner, the service and society. Autonomy is of extrinsic value to utilitarians, and is therefore non-essential, if the consequences are that by respecting the principle, less good is achieved than by not respecting it—in this case, autonomy should be overridden, as with the unnecessary rabies injection. Also, in Denise's case, if the general result of speeding up women's labours was to achieve safe delivery, staff satisfaction, and reduce the induction of a labour 'waiting list', then it would probably be accepted as creating 'greater good' and it would therefore be a suitable course of action.

There are two basic approaches to autonomy. The first is a broadly libertarian view; this assumes that anyone older than a toddler is autonomous, unless that toddler is mentally defective or possibly emotionally distraught. This is very much a generalization with no judging of capabilities, although it is considered that autonomy can be lost with age (e.g. senility). This approach suggests that a person's view must be accepted, even in the absence of an acceptable reason or rationality, thus allowing the freedom to make a mistake. This is the perspective often adopted by those on the libertarian end of the political spectrum and has been supported by philosophers such as Hume, Hobbes and Mill.

The second approach is more rigorous; rationality, reflection and clear judgement are essential factors and autonomy is considered to be a matter of degree rather than an 'all or nothing' capacity. The more rational and deliberate an individual's actions are, the more choice they are allowed; if these elements are weak or absent, then the question is whether or not the decisions should be overridden. Some supporters would consider that someone making decisions based on fear is using an irrational basis, therefore that person may not be acting autonomously. If that is the case, should decisions be made for that person, as in the case of the 'infamous', unconscious Jehovah's Witness requiring a blood transfusion? By this approach, individuals must show that they are doing the right thing for the right reasons, with no apparent 'freedom to make a mistake'. Supporters have included Plato and Rousseau, the latter believing that it is sometimes necessary to force people to be 'free'—either that or force them to make the choices appropriate to a rational, autonomous individual.

In this discussion there is concern for the autonomy of the women being cared for, and that of the health professionals concerned. The majority of these women are healthy, they are undergoing a natural—though not always problem free—process, one that involves physical, psychological and social change. Therefore the support to which they are entitled involves care within those three aspects, plus educational and, where appropriate, spiritual support. These aspects cannot be totally divorced from each other—there are areas of overlap. For instance, if a woman indicates a psychological problem, such as anxiety regarding pain in labour (perfectly understandable!), the midwife can discuss the various methods of pain relief available, teach her relaxation exercises and/or arrange for her to attend Preparation for Parenthood classes. In this way she has provided psychological support, education and an insight in to the physical support available. In so doing, the midwife will have created an awareness in the woman of possible choices. The degree of awareness created depends, among other things, on the woman's previous knowledge. From discussions with many midwives, as well as through personal experience, the author has determined that women appear generally more aware of their bodies and their labour options these days, possibly from the inclusion of health education programmes in schools and media coverage. Women from all walks of life have expectations of labour, themselves and their carers. It is by no means only the 'middle class' women who know what they want, although the level of expectation and understanding may be higher in some cases (Green et al., 1991). Nearly all women know at least what they do not want, they also want to be involved in decision making and give rational reasons for their decisions. This surely indicates that these women should be afforded the same respect for autonomy as any other rational person.

The midwife, in her everyday life, obviously has the same right to autonomy as any other person and this also applies to her working life. In their literature relating to admission to the Professional Register, the National Boards—part of the regulating system for nursing, midwifery and health visiting—state:

> *The Board considers that a midwife is a person who is qualified to take professional responsibility and to provide care as an* autonomous *practitioner for mothers during antenatal, intranatal and postnatal periods and for the neonates.*

(ENB, 1987)

This suggests that the midwife can use the knowledge, skills and attitudes acquired during training and subsequent practice, in order to achieve the best outcome, i.e. that required by the woman as well as the professionals. In practice, however, utilizing professional autonomy is very difficult; this is partly caused by the formulation of dogmatic unit policies and procedures. Many of these are very restrictive to the woman's freedom of apparent choice or movement, and to the midwife's practice. For instance, the policy of early rupture of membranes, as in the case study, is an invasive technique that is carried out, basically, 'just in case'. Coupled with this, it is also policy in many units to attach a fetal scalp electrode to the fetal head, or buttock, in order to monitor the heart rate. Generally, this means that the woman feels 'strapped' to her bed for the major part of her labour; it also means that the midwife is not being allowed to exercise her judgement with regard to the progress of labour or fetal condition (Robinson, 1990). This dogma even follows through to the immediate care of the woman after delivery. It would appear from discussion with midwives from various units—and with women who have experienced the care—that many units still have procedures that state that a bedbath be performed. If the woman–midwife partnership is functioning properly, then the woman could be offered the choice of a bedbath or shower, according to her wishes and the midwife's judgement regarding her condition.

Few professionals would argue against the formulation of policies and procedures for the safety of those receiving and giving care. Many do argue, however, that policies should be formulated by a more representative group of professionals. Inflexible, obstetric-orientated and litigation-fearing policies can create a conflict of interests between the obstetricians and midwives. Downe (1990a, b) poses the question:

> *... where does the midwife stand legally if a disaster occurs and she has not, on professional grounds, followed the hospital policy?*

From the employment point of view, if the policy was accepted by the health authority, she could have her employment terminated for failure to fulfil her contract. Professionally, however, a midwife cannot plead adherence to hospital policy if accused of misconduct, particularly if this is contrary to up-to-date professional knowledge. The 'Policies and Practices' committee (or whatever title it is given) should therefore be aware of up-to-date research, be able to evaluate it and be conversant with the needs and requests of the people they are serving. It would appear to be essential for clinical midwives, including a community representative, to be part of this decision-making body. It is not sufficient to have only the senior levels of staff represented—they are often too distant from the specific needs of both the women and the midwives. If this is considered at all, then a safe but flexible approach could be taken.

Doctors also have dual autonomy, as people and as practitioners. In their professional lives, they are in a position of authority and make decisions regarding the management of their patients' conditions and treatments. Ideally, in midwifery and obstetrics, this situation *should* only occur when a deviation from normal is detected as midwives are expert practitioners of normal midwifery. It is stated in the BMA *Handbook of Medical Ethics* (1986) that a midwife is:

> ... *permitted to deliver total care on her own responsibility to a woman and her baby during the antenatal, intranatal, postnatal and neonatal periods provided that complications are neither present nor arise.*

It also includes the fact that midwives must seek medical aid in the event of complications. Doctors are, therefore, covered to accept midwifery decisions in the absence of actual complications as the midwife will be accountable for her own decisions and actions.

Paternalism

It is possible that the midwife and/or doctor could be accused of behaving paternalistically in this case. To be paternalistic is to be very much like a Victorian father, the head of the household who knew what was best for everyone under his roof, particularly his children. Gert and Culver (1979) give the following definition.

> *A is acting paternalistically toward S if and only if A's behavior (correctly) indicates that A believes that:*

> *(1) his action is for S's good;*
> *(2) he is qualified to act on S's behalf;*
> *(3) his action involves violating a moral rule (or will require him to do so) with regard to S;*
> *(4) S's good justifies him acting on S's behalf independently of S's past, present or immediately forthcoming (free, informed) consent; and*
> *(5) S believes (perhaps falsely) that he (S) generally knows what is for his own good.*

In this definition, if the doctor is substituted for 'A', and Denise for 'S', one would suppose that he believes (1), (2) and (4); we know that (3) is correct as he was made aware of Denise's views and therefore—by acting without her consent—he has violated her autonomy. For her part, Denise feels that she knows what is best for herself. If we accept the definition, then this would confirm the view that the doctor is 'guilty' of paternalistic behaviour.

Paternalism can be on a large scale (as with governmental decisions) or a small scale (when dealing with individuals). In either case it can be coercive and it is possibly for this reason that antagonism towards it may develop. Examples of this large-scale concept could be fluoridation of water—where everyone in the area receives the service whether they want it or not—or the law relating to the use of seatbelts; a small scale example could be the decisions that some doctors might make, on behalf of a patient, without seeking or heeding their views. In each case this could be seen to be ignoring or overriding the autonomy of the individual, as in this case study.

Consent

... a voluntary, uncoerced decision, made by a sufficiently competent or autonomous person on the basis of adequate information and deliberation, to accept rather than reject some proposed course of action that will affect him or her.

(Gillon, 1986)

This definition indicates the relationship between autonomy and consent. If autonomy means being in control of your life, self-governing and self-ruled, then it is essential that the individual is at least a partner in any decision-making process that directly involves them. To be excluded from the process would mean that true consent has not been established.

Health care is one of the most important areas of life in which decisions must be made. People should not feel that they have removed their autonomy with their outdoor clothes, or the closing of an office door. If consent is not sought and gained before carrying out procedures, then the individual has not been allowed to fulfil the previously mentioned essentials of autonomy. In moral terms, therefore, it would seem correct to say that you cannot have one without the other: for consent to be requested, the person must be deemed autonomous; if the person is deemed autonomous then consent is essential, in order to preserve that autonomy.

In cases where the individuals are considered incompetent to make medical decisions—such as minors and the mentally incompetent—proxy consent may be obtained. Where minors are concerned, it is usual for parents to act in the 'best interests' of the child, but the court may intervene if it judges the course of action to be unreasonable. Where adult incompetents are concerned, decision making is achieved by 'substituted judgement'. In this case, the proxy decision maker considers him/herself in the position of the individual in question and decides what that person would want if competent to decide (Beauchamp and Childress, 1989). Where treatments may be controversial, doctor's may ask the opinion of the courts. The courts do not give actual consent, however, but if the case should come to court at a later date—possibly for negligence or battery—the actions and underlying concerns of the doctors would have been recorded (Dugdale, 1990; pers. comm.).

It is often assumed by the general public that they have to give their consent; this surely is not true consent, rather it is permission under assumed duress. They are often made to feel, by well-motivated health professionals, that they have no choice. There is always a choice: consent or refusal; sometimes there is also the possibility of compromise.

If people can give or withhold consent then they have a choice to make. If it is true that they always have a choice, how do they know which decision is the right one? Historically it was assumed that they could not know the answer, hence the paternalistic attitude of the medical, nursing and midwifery professions. More recently, however, there has been a move towards gaining informed consent, brought about to some extent by certain legal cases at home and abroad. This is achieved by giving the 'patients' as much information as they need, in understandable terms, in order for them to view their own situation accurately and reach their own decision. A number of court cases have held that the giving of adequate information, prior to requesting consent to procedures, is part of the duty of care—it cannot, therefore, be omitted without a breach of that duty being committed (Dimond, 1990).

APPLYING THE THEORIES

A utilitarian view

Denise has been shown to be an autonomous person; as such she is entitled to make decisions regarding her care. She did this by writing a birthplan, a plan she wanted to follow unless circumstances called for joint discussion, possibly resulting in a change in the decisions she had made. By following the plan, the professionals would have preserved Denise's feeling of self-control and her positive view of her experience by observing autonomy. They may also have prevented the increase in pain. They would certainly have prevented the letter of complaint, with professional harmony and integrity being maintained. By not following the plan, there was no observance of autonomy, a trespass against the person was committed, professional disharmony might continue—particularly in view of the letter of complaint—and an unnecessary investigative process would be time-consuming. The balance would appear to be in favour of observing the client's wishes.

A deontological view

Both professionals have duties to this client, however, it is the midwife's actions that are being considered. According to the list on page 29 she had a number of duties to her client: fidelity (which includes advocacy and truth-telling), beneficence and nonmaleficence particularly. These duties must be observed, therefore this theory upholds the use of this particular plan.

SUGGESTED READING REGARDING AUTONOMY AND CONSENT

Beauchamp, T.L. and Childress, J.F. (1989) *Principles of Biomedical Ethics*, 3rd edn, Oxford University Press, Oxford.

Dimond, B. (1990) *Legal Aspects of Nursing*, Prentice Hall, London.

Dworkin, G. (1988) *The Theory and Practice of Autonomy*, Cambridge University Press, Cambridge.

Faulder, C. (1985) *Whose Body Is It?* Virago Press, London.

Johnson, A.G. (1990) *Pathways in Medical Ethics*, Edward Arnold, London, Chapter 8.

Lee, S. (1990) Whose consent?, in *Ethics in Reproductive Medicine* (eds D.R. Bromham *et al.*), Manchester University Press, Manchester.

Robinson, S. (1990) The role of the midwife: Opportunities and constraints, in *Effective Care in Pregnancy and Childbirth Volume 1* (eds I. Chalmers *et al.*), Oxford University Press, Oxford, Chapter 10.

SUGGESTED READING REGARDING ARTIFICIAL RUPTURE OF THE MEMBRANES

Flint, C. (1990) Artificial rupture of the membranes: Time to think again? *Obs. Gyn. Product News* (Autumn).

Fraser, W.D. *et al.* (1991) A randomized controlled trial of early amniotomy. *Br. J. Obs. Gyn.* (January), **98**, 84 (abstract).

Henderson, C. (1990) Artificial rupture of the membranes, in *Midwifery Practice—Intrapartum care* (eds J. Alexander *et al.*), Macmillan Educational, London.

NCT (1989) *Rupture of the Membranes in Labour*.

REFERENCES

Entries marked '*' are bibliographical entries rather than—or as well as—references.

*Bakhurst, D. (1992) On lying and deceiving. *J. Med. Ethics*, **18**, 63–66.

*Beauchamp, T.L. and Childress, J.F. (1989) *Principles of Biomedical Ethics*, 3rd edn, Oxford University Press, Oxford, pp.71–72.

Benjamin, M. and Curtis, J. (1986) *Ethics in Nursing*, 2nd edn, Oxford University Press, Oxford, p.21.

*BMA (1986) *The Handbook of Medical Ethics*, Cambridge University Press, Cambridge, pp.19, 38.

*Brazier, M. (1987) *Medicine, Patients and the Law*, Penguin Books, Middlesex, p.56.

Buchanan, A. (1978) Medical paternalism, in *The Theory and Practice of Autonomy* (ed. G. Dworkin), Cambridge University Press, Cambridge, p.122.

*Campbell, A.V. (1984) *Moral Dilemmas in Medicine*, 3rd edn, Churchill Livingstone, London.

*Carter, R. (1977) Justifying paternalism. *Canadian J. Philos.*, **7**, 139–140.

*Chamberlain, G. and Orr, C. (eds)(1990) *How to Avoid Medico-Legal Problems in Obstetrics and Gynaecology*, The Chameleon Press, London.

*Dimond, B. (1990) *Legal Aspects of Nursing*, Prentice Hall, London, pp.88–89, 93.

Downe, S. (1990a) We must mean what we say. *Nursing Times*, **85**(20), 25.

Downe, S. (1990b) Conflict of interests. *Nursing Times*, **86**(47), 14.

*Downie, R.S. and Calman, K.C. (1987) *Healthy Respect—Ethics in health care*, Faber and Faber,London, Chapters 4 and 6, p.51.

Dunn, P.M. (1978) Problems Associated With Foetal Monitoring During Labour. *Proceedings of the 6th European Congress on Perinatal Medicine*, pp.270–274.

Dworkin, G. (1988) *The Theory and Practice of Autonomy*, Cambridge University Press, Cambridge, p.121.

ENB (1987) *Course Leading to Part 10 of the Professional Register—Registered Midwife*, p.2.

*Faulder, C. (1985) *Whose Body Is It?* Virago Press, London, pp.29–30, 128.

Flint, C. (1987) Midwives' judgement. *Nursing Times* (4 March), 39.

*Flint, C. (1990) Artificial rupture of the membranes: Time to think again? *Obs. Gyn. Product News* (Autumn), 27–28.

*Fraser, W.D. *et al.* (1991) A randomized controlled trial of early amniotomy. *Br. J. Obs. Gyn.* (January), **98**, 84 (abstract).

Gabbe, S.G. *et al.* (1976) Umbilical cord compression associated with amniotomy: laboratory observations. *Am. J. Obs. Gyn.*, **126**(3), 353–355.

Gert, B. and Culver, C.M. (1979) The justification of paternalism, in *Medicine and Moral Philosophy—Readings from philosophy and public affairs*, Princeton University Press, p.199.

*Gillett, G.R. (1989) Informed consent and moral integrity. *J. Med. Ethics*, **15**, 117–123.

*Gillon, R. (1986) *Philosophical Medical Ethics*, Wiley and Sons, Chichester, Chapters 10 and 18, pp.113, 166.

*GMC (1987) *Professional Conduct and Discipline: Fitness to practice.*

*Gorovitz, S. (1990) Informed consent, in *Ethics in Reproductive Medicine* (eds D.R. Bromham *et al.*), Manchester University Press, Manchester, pp.228–235.

Green, J.M. *et al.* (1991) Expectations, experiences and psychological outcomes of childbirth: A prospective study of 825 women. *Birth*, **17**(1), 15–24.

*Henderson, C. (1990) Artificial rupture of the membranes, in *Midwifery Practice— Intrapartum care* (eds J. Alexander *et al.*), Macmillan Educational, London, pp.46, 52.

*Johnson, A.G. (1990) *Pathways in Medical Ethics*, Edward Arnold, London, Chapter 8.

*Lee, S. (1990) Whose consent?, in *Ethics in Reproductive Medicine* (eds D.R. Bromham *et al.*), Manchester University Press, Manchester, pp.236–261.

*Lilford, R. and Thornton, J. (1990) In *Ethics in Reproductive Medicine* (eds D.R. Bromham *et al.*), Manchester University Press, Manchester, pp.211–227.

*Lockwood, M. (ed.)(1985) *Moral Dilemmas in Modern Medicine*, Oxford University Press, Oxford, Chapter 5.

Mason, J.K. and McCall Smith, R.A. (1987) *Law and Medical Ethics*, Butterworths, London, p.149.

*NCT (1989) *Rupture of the Membranes in Labour*, pp.32, 35, 36–37, 41.

RCM *Practical Guidance for Midwives Facing Ethical or Moral Dilemmas*, London.

*Robinson, S. *et al.* (1983) *A Study of the Role and Responsibilities of the Midwife*, University of London, pp.329–331.

Robinson, S. (1990) The role of the midwife: Opportunities and constraints, in *Effective Care in Pregnancy and Childbirth Volume 1* (eds I. Chalmers *et al.*), Oxford University Press, Oxford, Chapter 10, pp.162–180.

Smythe, C.N. (1974) Biomechanics and Human Parturition. *Proc. Roy. Soc. Med.*, **67**, 189–193.

UKCC (1989) *Exercising Accountability*, pp.10–11.

WHO (1985) Appropriate technology for birth, in *MIDIRS Information Pack No.5* (August 1986).

5.

SCREENING FOR FETAL ABNORMALITY

CASE STUDY

Joyce is 37 years old. She and her husband Simon have been informed that she is pregnant, following two spontaneous abortions (miscarriages) in the last two years—one was at 8 weeks, the other at 12 weeks. In view of Joyce's age it has been suggested that screening for genetic abnormality could be performed, either by chorionic villus sampling or amniocentesis. Joyce is generally opposed to abortion but would consider it for major fetal abnormality. Simon has no firm opinion regarding abortion but has said in the past that he could not cope with a handicapped child.

QUESTIONS FOR CONSIDERATION BY THE READER

1. Should fetal screening be encouraged by midwives?

2. Would it be right to leave Joyce and Simon to choose for themselves which procedure to follow?

3. What possible options are open to Joyce and Simon if the fetus is discovered to have an abnormality?

4. Is fetal screening always a positive action?

5. What is the role of the midwife where the results indicate abnormality?

Question 1. Should fetal screening be encouraged by midwives?

This is a general question and does not relate to any particular group of women, therefore we are looking at all fetal screening. Should midwives be advising all women to be screened? And if so, for which conditions? If resources were unlimited, would all women be encouraged to be tested for all detectable abnormality? It is necessary that readers consider this question carefully as, when using this case study with student midwives, the author found that they tended to interpret it as 'Is screening a good idea?' which is a very different question.

It creates an opening to consider the general principles of screening rather than the specific problems relating to autonomy and eugenics. The question has not been altered as the error itself, if it is made, can be used as a good learning point.

Screening is generally the preliminary step towards the detection of disorders that may require further investigation. It can be used where specific disorders are anticipated in high-risk individuals—e.g. genetic disorders—or it can be used with a large sample of the population, as is carried out for rubella immunity in pregnancy. In itself it is not diagnosis. Diagnosis is the actual identification of a disease/disorder by use of scientific means, part of which would include the results of screening (Mosby, 1986). These terms are therefore not interchangeable.

To promote uptake of the tests suggests persuading women that they ought to opt for what is available. This would surely be a paternalistic approach (as discussed in the case study 'Autonomy and consent'). If it is accepted that the woman's autonomy is important, and consent is required, then professionals cannot indulge in paternalism. It would be more appropriate to provide sufficient written and verbal information in terms understood by the public. This information should include what the test is for, what it entails, the possible results and their accuracy, any risks involved and the choices open to the woman in the event of abnormality—or appropriate sex for the inheritance of the disease in question—being detected. Proper counselling facilities should be made available in order to give the results of the test, whether good or bad. This would allow the woman and her partner to discuss their feelings and make their own decisions if necessary.

It would be fair to say—through the author's own observations and those reported to her—that gaining informed consent to routine screening procedures rarely occurs. There will undoubtedly be some practitioners—midwives and doctors—in some hospitals or communities who give all the information required and then give the woman an opportunity to discuss her views and feelings before she makes her decision, but they are few and far between. How many practitioners, for instance, tell mothers what blood tests will be performed, and actually obtain consent? Although midwives seem to be improving in this area, it is still too frequent an occurrence to hear statements such as:

We need to take some blood today.

At which point the practitioner would accept the implied consent of the woman raising her sleeve and offering her arm (Dimond, 1990). Sometimes the statement will be expanded to:

... to find out your blood group and whether you are anaemic... .

Too often one hears:

> We would like to take some blood today. The tests carried out are to find
> out what your blood group is, whether you are anaemic and immune to
> rubella. It is also tested for syphilis, hepatitis B and—if appropriate—
> sickle cell anaemia. Would you like to ask any questions about these tests
> and would you be happy to have them done? (Or words to that effect.)

The same can be said of the next routine test offered, the alpha-feto protein
(AFP) test. When it first became available, women were told about it and asked
if they would want their pregnancy terminated if the test indicated that the fetus
had a neural tube defect. If they said 'Yes', blood was taken. There are arguments
that could be raised about that, particularly the fact that they had to be in favour
of termination on receipt of a positive result before they were offered the test.
In 1987, the King's Fund Forum Consensus Statement on 'Screening for Fetal
and Genetic Abnormality' included:

> A woman's access to a screening or diagnostic test should be inde-
> pendent of any decision she may make about the continuation of the
> pregnancy.

This would seem morally correct but the counselling that occurred in the initial
stages of offering the test was at least better than that offered in many cases
today. Women were given more information on the test and the possible outcomes than they are now. All too often one hears of women being asked if they
want 'the spina bifida test' or 'the blood test to see if the baby's alright'.
Sometimes they are not really asked at all, it is merely assumed that they want
it and the same procedure occurs as previously described. This would not
appear to be the case with the more invasive techniques of chorionic villus sampling, amniocentesis and fetal blood sampling where proper counselling usually
takes place. Verbal comment from various sources suggests that some doctors
will only offer these techniques to women who would continue on to termination, and that some women have had 'very high' AFP results and have been
advised to terminate their pregnancies without any further investigation, only to
find that having refused abortion their babies were normal; they had been highly
stressed throughout the rest of their pregnancies.

Question 2. Would it be right to leave Joyce and Simon to choose for themselves which procedure to follow?

This concerns the autonomy of the couple—whether they should be given all information with no bias and left to make a decision alone, or be advised by midwives and doctors (an element of paternalism). They would need to know the advantages and disadvantages of both tests, information about which can be found in 'Further discussion'.

Question 3. What possible options are open to Joyce and Simon if the fetus is discovered to have an abnormality?

In this question it is suggested that one presumes that Joyce chose to undergo one of the tests and an abnormality was discovered. It is not known which test, therefore it is not known at what gestation the options are finally being faced. Gestation is irrelevant to the options available though it may be relevant in the decision-making process and it is certainly relevant to the method of abortion should this be the chosen outcome. The options that are available to this couple are abortion, fostering/adoption or parenting the child themselves.

In the case study it is stated that Joyce would consider abortion if the fetus had a major abnormality, but it is often difficult to ascertain what is considered 'major'. Usually this would include the so-called 'monsters'—often those where twinning is incomplete, and cases of neural tube defect. For some people it would also include Down's syndrome, for others it would not. This dilemma possibly arises from the difficulty in prediction of the degree of mental and physical abnormality with which the baby may be born—this would not be established by the test. At one time it was only the mental incapacity associated with the condition of which lay-people were aware, and these days so much more can be done to compensate for this. It is stated that Simon has no definite feelings about abortion, but he may have firm views about certain handicaps and conditions. He had mentioned this in the past, therefore Joyce would proba- bly have his assistance in making a decision, rather than his leaving it up to her. The problem that could arise, however, is that Simon may view the abnormality as automatically being an indication for abortion whereas Joyce might not. This could lead to friction within their partnership, possibly leading to resentment by one or other partner.

It must be a very difficult decision for most couples to make. Perhaps it is a little easier in the first trimester, but with a history of spontaneous abortions and increasing parental age (the woman in particular) there may be the concern that aborting this pregnancy could commit them to childlessness. This could occur from decreased fertility or further spontaneous abortion; it could also be that from fear of conceiving another abnormal fetus they would choose to be childless, however painful the decision. It is possible that they would find this preferable to having a handicapped child, unlike Harris' (1990) suggestion:

> *If children are wanted, it is better to have healthy children than to have handicapped children where these are alternatives, and it is better to have handicapped children than no children at all.*

Although decisions rest with the couple alone, it would be a mistake to assume that outside influences are ignored. Apart from listening to professional points of view, couples will often consider the opinions of family and friends. If they feel that their child would be poorly received then this might aid their decision to abort the fetus. On the other hand, if they feel that there would be positive and supportive reaction, then they may be able to cope with the possible trials ahead. Their general socialization, from childhood onwards, would also influence their decision-making: education; religious beliefs; and media portrayal of handicaps in general. Down's syndrome has fared particularly well since the MENCAP campaign of the late 1970s and early 1980s, with society being better educated to accept people with this disorder.

It could be argued that Joyce and Simon—depending on the geneticist's findings—may have grounds for seeking adoption rather than embarking on another pregnancy but this is not realistic. Joyce is already older than most adoption agencies' age limit for adopting normal babies/children and there are very few babies for adoption anyway. Agencies are often prepared to consider older couples for those children who are 'hard to place' (such as the handicapped) but this would obviously be inappropriate in this case. Their only chance would be to apply to an agency where their ages were accepted and try to adopt an older child. Here too the influence of family and friends can be very strong. The gestation may be one of the most significant factors. If they chose to wait for the amniocentesis, for the reasons outlined earlier, they may find that to decide on abortion when the pregnancy is nearly half-way through—and the fetus has been seen on a scanner screen—is much more difficult than they might have predicted, especially for Joyce. Hence the reason for offering early diagnostic tests regardless of parental feelings regarding abortion.

If they feel they cannot opt for abortion for this condition at the later gestation but also cannot face the problems of parenting a handicapped child, then perhaps they would consider placing the child for adoption. It is not easy to place such babies but there are more families now who are willing to undertake this task. If they are not certain about this course of action but are still unable to opt for abortion, then it is possible that a foster family may be found until they are able to reach a decision. Institutional life is the alternative if adoption and fostering fail.

It is possible that they will decide to continue with the pregnancy and prepare themselves for what is to come. This would include discussions with a geneticist regarding the expected degree of abnormality, a paediatrician regarding possible defects and their treatment and, if the condition is Down's syndrome, a visit to an assessment centre. At the centre they would see children of various ages and stages of development playing with a variety of educational toys, apparently no different from other children. They would have the opportunity to talk to other parents as well as professionals who would discuss the suggested plans for after their baby is born. Some women choose to be tested with no intention of having an abortion—they may be choosing to know of any detectable handicap in order to grieve for the loss of 'what might have been', giving better opportunity for bonding after delivery. Also, it gives time to prepare for what is facing them and how they are going to cope with it.

It should be remembered that we do not make decisions in a vacuum. We are often influenced and constrained by the views of others. Family and friends were previously mentioned in this respect but society in general imposes opinions, particularly (in this case) with regard to the perceived value of the lives of handicapped people. These opinions are often voiced through the media but they are also expressed verbally and non-verbally in streets, shops and other public places. In some cases comments are made during conversations, in others it may be the sight of a handicapped child or adult that causes comment or facial expression. The attitudes exhibited range from pity, through a variety of others, to repulsion. The knowledge that this will undoubtedly occur at some time will be in the minds of many people facing this type of decision, with consideration of whether they can cope with either extreme.

Society's views of screening tests for fetal abnormality could be creating a 'roller-coaster' effect. The test is performed, an abnormality is discovered, therefore termination of pregnancy is accepted or even expected. This is based on the perceived quality of life as opposed to the value of life. We live in a 'disposable' age: if something is imperfect it is thrown away and replaced. It is possible this could eventually happen with minor fetal defects. Society may even develop expectations that all 'at risk' women should be tested, with no freedom of choice.

Whatever Joyce and Simon opt for, they would be advised to seek genetic counselling for future pregnancies, especially in view of the previous spontaneous abortions.

Question 4. Is fetal screening always a positive action?

It is necessary to consider fetal screening more generally again in question 4. Green (1990), through the Galton Institute, has produced an Occasional Paper *Calming or Harming? A critical review of psychological effects of fetal diagnosis on pregnant women*. The studies that were reviewed indicated what most people would have expected:

In all cases there is the potential both to allay anxiety and to create it.

The intention of the tests is to diagnose abnormality as well as confirm the absence of some abnormalities. The author would suggest, however, that most women are expecting the latter when they first agree to the tests. Green noted, from the studies, that genetic counselling had little effect on the decisions regarding tests or abortion. However, there were things that did have effect, not on the decisions but on the emotional state of the women. In some cases it was the false positive results, in others the length of waiting time that made women anxious. In many cases it was the attitude or non-communication of the operator, particularly with ultrasound scanning. In some UK hospitals it is the policy that ultrasound scanner operators—unless it is the doctors themselves—are not allowed to make comments on the scan, whether abnormality is detected or not. This must also create tension for the operators. Simply offering the test casts doubt on the fetal condition; this must surely be very stressful for most women, particularly if they do not consider themselves to be at risk. For those whose results are abnormal, the stress is unavoidable at some stage, but those who receive normal results will have had anxiety created that may not be easily relieved. Some of these women may carry their anxiety through labour and into the postnatal period even though their babies appear normal, giving cause for concern to their relatives and to the professionals caring for them.

On the other hand, many women appear to accept normal AFP results as meaning *everything* is normal. The discovery of another abnormality can therefore be devastating. It could be suggested that, in these cases, these tests are inadvertently giving a false expectation with regard to fetal normality.

Near the beginning of this discussion (in the list of those 'at risk') cases such as rubella and toxoplasmosis contacts were included. It was interesting to see that immediately following a television programme about the latter, women started to demand that their antenatal clinics should offer the test. It is being offered more widely now, with a campaign underway to offer it routinely, as in France. The fact that it is now offered in some places indicates that public pressure can create changes. Once these women are tested and confirmed as having the disease, they can be treated, if identified early enough.

Unfortunately this is not the case for those with rubella. The situation then arises where women/couples must decide for or against abortion with no confirmation of whether or not the fetus is affected. Similar circumstances can arise with sex-linked diseases: having determined, for instance, that the fetus is male, it may be that there is a 1:4 chance of the fetus being affected. Decisions to abort could therefore result in normal, unaffected foetuses being terminated, whereas decisions to continue with the pregnancies could result in babies being born with severe handicaps or life-threatening disorders.

In the wider social and political context, it could also be asked whether it is right to indulge in fetal screening and whether the changes in the NHS—purchasing and providing—will make any difference. Screening could be considered a step towards creating a 'master race', especially as technology advances and more diseases and conditions can be detected. Even with present abilities, we could be seen to be giving society a false expectation of total perfection every time. It should also be questioned as to whether or not screening and selective abortion may cause society to lose experience in caring and 'making way' for less fortunate people.

Question 5. What is the role of the midwife where the results indicate abnormality?

The midwife's role is multi-facetted. Here is one way of interpreting the role in relation to this question.

PRACTITIONER It may be the midwife who is giving Joyce/the couple the results. She should not lie to her clients and therefore she may be forced to answer their queries regarding the results, even if this is not the usual practice in her area. Regardless of the decision that is made, the midwife must continue to care for Joyce in an appropriate manner until the end of her pregnancy (at whatever stage this occurs). It would depend on local policies and the couple's views as to how much involvement she would have following a termination of pregnancy.

COUNSELLOR Having given Joyce the results (or following the doctor's undertaking of the task) the midwife needs to be available to listen to her and/or Simon. They are facing a major decision in their lives, in circumstances where they are probably too stressed to think as clearly as they might normally when making decisions. They may need someone to give them time to verbalize their thoughts and fears. Often a midwife is selected for this purpose, particularly if a good rapport has been established.

ADVISOR She cannot tell the couple what they should do but she can advise them on possible options and the various personnel who can further advise or answer questions.

FRIEND This couple—and Joyce in particular—will require a lot of support, not only during the decision-making process but also following whichever course of action they choose to take. A midwife is in the position of being able to give that support without being judgemental. For this reason she will possibly seem more of a friend than their actual friends at this time.

ADVOCATE It is possible that during this very unsettling time Joyce may need someone to help her state her case. This could involve other professionals or members of Joyce's family, possibly even Simon.

EDUCATOR This could involve further explanations about the initial test(s) and results, or it could entail explanations of what is to come, whether she chooses abortion or continuance of the pregnancy. If she chooses to continue, then all the usual education will also be required.

FURTHER DISCUSSION

Modern technology has provided society with the opportunity of diagnosing a pregnancy before the woman has missed her first menstrual period, a very different picture to 20 years ago when women waited until at least two missed periods before seeking confirmation of pregnancy. This earlier confirmation (coupled with advanced technology) provides greater opportunity for investigating the state of the fetus, should this be required.

It would seem reasonable to determine what is meant by 'fetal screening'. It sounds as though all foetuses are checked, from head to toe, inside and out, to detect any possible abnormality. This is obviously not the case—at least it is obvious to those who have regular dealings with such matters, but what about the general public? It is possible that they expect more of technology and the Health Service than is actually available. This point will be discussed later on but meanwhile the author will accept the definition of screening provided by Cuckle and Wald (1984) as:

> ... the identification, among apparently healthy individuals, of those who are sufficiently at risk of a specific disorder to justify a subsequent diagnostic test or procedure, or in certain circumstances, direct preventive action.

There are basically two types of fetal screening. The first deals with the routine screening offered to all mothers who attend clinics early enough for it to be carried out. The second relates to the 'at risk' woman, whose fetus/baby is at greater risk of genetic disorders or congenital abnormality. This would include:

• Those who have previously had babies with certain abnormalities.
• Where there is a family history of such problems.
• Where either the woman or her partner have an inheritable disease or one that could create other abnormalities in the baby, such as diabetes mellitus.
• Where the woman has contracted diseases such as rubella or toxoplasmosis during early pregnancy.
• Where the woman is 35 years old or older (as with Joyce) when it is considered more likely that chromosomal abnormality could occur.

Although antenatal screening tests are specific, they do not always directly screen the fetus. Some of them test the woman for conditions that could adversely affect her or her fetus in pregnancy, labour or infancy/childhood. Testing for human immunodeficiency virus status could be included in this category. Although it is not routine for all women to be tested, midwives must be

aware that it is carried out in some cases. Women who are considered, by themselves or the professionals in attendance to be 'at risk' can be offered the
opportunity of being tested with no obligation to accept. Also, there is national
epidemiological research in process, which is designed to indicate the spread of
the disease through various sections of the community:

> *i.e. unlinked, anonymous prevalence data testing...*
> (Pratt, 1991)

At a number of hospitals throughout the UK, women attending antenatal clinics
are being tested. As the intention is not to discover which individuals are
human immunodeficiency virus positive, the testing is anonymous; this means
that although they know they are being tested, those who are 'positive' will not
be informed. There is obviously much to debate on this issue but it will not be
continued here.

Other tests are specific to fetal condition. These include ultrasound scanning, AFP estimation, fetal blood sampling, chorionic villus sampling and
amniocentesis.

Chorionic villus sampling

This technique is usually carried out between 8 and 11 weeks of pregnancy,
with the aid of ultrasound scanning. Early diagnosis of pregnancy is, therefore,
essential for this test to be of maximum benefit. It can be performed vaginally,
through the uterine cervix, or abdominally, involving the extraction of a sample
of the chorionic villi (the tree-like projections of trophoblast which burrow into
the decidua to form the placenta). This test is used to detect:

• Chromosomal abnormalities such as Down's syndrome.
• Inborn errors of metabolism.
• The sex (where sex-linked diseases are in question).
• To enable DNA analysis (for cystic fibrosis, etc.).

It cannot detect structural abnormalities.

There are a number of advantages to this test, the most important perhaps being
that the woman has not progressed far into her pregnancy before she either has
her initial fears confirmed or allayed. With a 2% risk of spontaneous abortion
attached to the transabdominal procedure—and a higher rate associated with
the transcervical route (Birmingham Maternity Hospital, 1989)—it might
therefore be generally preferable to take that risk early rather than later in the
pregnancy.

If the test results are to prove unfavourable then early testing can be preferable in a number of ways. For instance, she may not want family, friends and
neighbours to know that she is pregnant in case she chooses to have an abortion.

At this stage it would not be obvious to others and, as the fetal cells are still undergoing rapid reproduction, results only take a few days. Also, although it is still her 'baby', she is less likely to have become familiar with it, as fetal movements and abdominal growth would not yet be experienced. At this early stage of pregnancy, if abortion is her choice of action, she would be able to undergo the routine procedure for early termination of pregnancy with a general anaesthetic, as the uterus would still be a pelvic organ and the conceptus would be small enough to be aborted in theatre.

There are also disadvantages. As previously mentioned, there is a risk of procedure-related abortion (Lilford and Thornton, 1990). In Joyce's case this could be of particular concern in view of her history of two spontaneous abortions. It is important to remember that the results could be favourable, but having ruled out the disorders which chorionic villus sampling would have disclosed, there is still no guarantee that the fetus does not have a neural tube defect or other structural abnormality.

Another possible disadvantage is that, while the test may be performed in order to diagnose or rule out certain chromosomal disorders, it is possible that it could detect something that was not previously considered. This could create a dilemma for the doctors, particularly if the prognosis is unknown or there is a good chance that the anomaly will not produce a major problem, such as an extra Y chromosome (Richards, 1988; Beauchamp and Childress, 1989). The author is not suggesting that Richards' hypothetical thoughts should be adopted:

Perhaps we need to discipline ourselves to ignore information that arrives by serendipity.

Rather, it is being highlighted that unless good counselling has taken place regarding this possibility, the woman/couple may not be prepared for the actual findings.

Amniocentesis

This is also an invasive procedure, performed with the aid of ultrasound scanning, whereby approximately 20 ml of amniotic fluid is withdrawn from around the fetus. It is performed abdominally and cannot be performed until the uterus has risen into the abdominal cavity; also, there must be sufficient fluid present for the sample to be taken without causing too great a fluid loss. It is usually carried out between the 14th and 18th weeks of pregnancy. As fetal cell reproduction is much slower at this time, it is necessary for the cells to be cultured and this usually takes two weeks but may take up to three.

During the examination of the chromosomes, the gender of the fetus is determined. In some health authorities the policy is to withhold this information unless this was the reason for the investigation, and to this end it is omitted from the specimen result sheet. The reason for this would appear to be that doctors are concerned that the gender of the fetus may play too large a role in the decision-making process. This surely is a paternalistic action, as whatever the test indicates, the woman, having consented to the test, is entitled to know the full results. Those who do not wish to know the sex of their children before they are born, have the right to request that they remain in ignorance of it. Amniocentesis can be used to detect the same abnormalities as chorionic villus sampling, with the added advantage of detecting AFP, which may indicate neural tube defect, therefore completing all the initial tests at one time. The other advantage associated with this method of testing, may be that a woman in Joyce's position might feel that the pregnancy is more secure at this later stage, perhaps depending on the fact that there is less risk of procedure-related abortion, which Lilford and Thornton (1990) estimate as being 0.5%. Although experience has created a safer technique, there is still the risk of injury to the fetus at the time of the test, and from removal of too much fluid, as well as from procedure-related abortion. It should also be remembered that there is the possibility of discovering something that was not being sought (as discussed under chorionic villus sampling).

There are also a number of disadvantages to this procedure, generally related to the stage of pregnancy. The pregnancy is well established and is also visible to family, friends and neighbours. In fact, the woman may well feel fetal movements by the time she receives the results, perhaps creating more of a dilemma for her if the results indicate abnormality. The other disadvantage related to gestation is the required method of termination—this involves the endurance of an induced labour and therefore the need to consider adequate pain relief and professional support.

The place of care of late termination is of great concern to many practitioners. Most agree that the delivery suite is preferable to a gynaecological ward, but many dilemmas are created by this, which will not be discussed here.

The effects of late testing

The delay in receiving the results, following the later gestation at which the test is performed, has always been a major concern, with the legal limit for abortion having been 28 weeks' gestation. The *Abortion Act 1967* (as amended), however, has inadvertently allowed for this dilemma as there is no longer a time limit for abortions of this nature. It is no longer legal to abort a fetus after the 24th completed week of pregnancy, except in cases where the life of the woman is in jeopardy or the baby would be seriously mentally or physically handicapped. Many advocates of abortion for gross fetal abnormality will be pleased that there is flexibility for such cases but they may be distressed to consider termination of pregnancy up to and including the expected date of delivery.

It is interesting to note Baroness Cox's (1991) observations since the Act was passed:

> Britain is the only country in Europe to have legalised abortion up to birth, and in my experience, many people up and down the land did not realise what was happening. Indeed, one of the bishops in the debate courageously admitted that he had not fully understood the implications of the new law: he had not realised the difference between termination of pregnancy in which every effort is made to save a viable baby, and a late abortion, in which the object of the exercise is to destroy a viable baby.

It is difficult to contemplate the possible outcomes of the change in the Act:

> In one delivery room there could be a baby, born alive at twenty four weeks of pregnancy following a preterm labour, where vigorous attempts are made to keep him/her alive. The prognosis would be unknown, but all efforts would be made in the knowledge that the technology exists to give him the best possible chance of survival.
>
> In another room, a woman is being prepared for theatre at thirty weeks gestation, where the baby will probably undergo similar care (to the first one) following 'termination' of the pregnancy for severe maternal illness. This woman would probably be most concerned that her baby should not be sacrificed for her, yet she would know that she effectively had no real choice if she wanted to survive.
>
> In a third room, yet another woman is enduring labour, perhaps at thirty-two weeks gestation, where the intention is for the fetus not to survive. This would be the case in a labour concerning a previously undiagnosed anencephalic fetus, as it would be incompatible with sustained life, but we would expect that many other fetuses with various abnormalities, such as Down's Syndrome, would survive labour and delivery and would usually be capable of sustained independent life. In this case the fetus would have been killed in utero, possibly by injecting potassium chloride into/close to the fetal heart.
>
> (Cole and Duddington, 1990)

Is late abortion any different, in principle, to the intentions of the late Dr Leonard Arthur who was accused (and acquitted):

> ... of the attempted murder of a newborn infant with Down's syndrome for whom he had prescribed dihydrocodeine and 'nursing care only' after the baby had been rejected by his mother.
>
> (Gillon, 1986)

Although there would have been opposing views put forward by various individuals, Kuhse and Singer (1985) acknowledge that the majority of the British public—86% according to a BBC poll—were in favour of his acquittal.

Fagot-Largeault (1990) stated that:

Legal distinctions are also in agreement with the common intuition that the termination of a defective fetus is morally more acceptable than the termination of a healthy fetus of the same age.

Abortion

Abortion is a very sensitive subject that can stimulate very passionate responses across the spectrum of society. The intention here is to indicate some of the major points of the argument, not to enter the actual abortion debate. One view is that an embryo is a human life from conception and all human life must be preserved. An opposing view is that—regardless of the status of the embryo/fetus—the woman has the right to determine what happens to her own body, including the decision regarding the termination of a pregnancy. There are a number of points of view that come between—or encompass part of—these opposing views and there are various issues involved. These include consideration of when life begins, the value of that life and the notion of 'personhood' and potential (Morgan and Lee, 1991). There is then the consideration of the rights of the fetus, whether it has any and how they fit in with the rights of the woman (see 'Maternal versus fetal rights').

Another question raised by some is that of fathers' rights. There have been occasional challenges, such as the Paton case in 1978 (Kenny, 1986) and one in Maryland, USA, (Gallagher, 1984), but no challenge has been upheld legally. The Abortion Act 1967 (as amended) will continue to be a major issue in the abortion debate, not only because of the differing views on abortion itself but also because of the implications of the removal of the time limit for certain categories, as previously indicated.

There is another aspect to consider here: the views of the carers. It can be very distressing for staff to be involved in the care of women who may—for whatever reason—be opting for abortion. Midwives should be fully aware of their own views, ensuring that they give unbiased information in a non-judgemental manner. They have a duty to care for each woman but they are not expected to compromise themselves. Any midwife who has a conscientious objection to abortion should put this in writing to her manager; she will then be excused from care during the actual abortion procedure but not from pre- and post-procedure care. However, in the case of an emergency occurring she would be expected to carry out whatever care is required (HMSO, 1967, *Abortion Act 1967*, amended).

APPLYING THE THEORIES

A utilitarian view of screening

Screening creates the possibility of detecting abnormality. Such detection allows for possible correction of the problem, for abortion or for preparation of the parents and staff. Where correction or abortion are concerned, this prevents the need for long-term provision of care, which is often expensive (financially and emotionally). Following any of these options, supportive services will be needed for the parents. If screening is not carried out, then many more abnormal babies would be born to women who have not been prepared. Those babies who survive could create a large drain on health and social services. It is possible that the parents would reject their babies or require long-term institutionalized care. Whatever the parental response, supportive services would be needed. The balance of consequences, for the utilitarian, would appear to lie in favour of screening with a view to correction or abortion.

A deontological view of screening

Deontology has a strong religious basis, with particular regard to the sanctity of life. In view of this, it would seem unlikely that deontologists would be in favour of screening with a view to abortion. However, they may well be in favour of preparation and certain forms of correction.

SUGGESTED READING

Cole, A.P.and Duddington, J.G. (1990) Altered grounds for abortion? *Lancet*, **336**(8730), 22–29 December.

Fagot-Largeault, A. (1990) The notion of the potential human being, in *Philosophical Ethics in Reproductive Medicine* (ed. Bromham *et al.*), Manchester University Press, Manchester.

Green, J.M. (1990) *Calming or harming?* Occasional Papers, 2nd Series, No 2., Galton Institute.

HMSO (1990) *Abortion (Amendment) Act 1990*, HMSO, London.

Richards, M.P.M. (1989) Social and ethical problems of fetal diagnosis and screening. *J. Reproduct. Infant Psychol.*, **7**, 171–185.

REFERENCES

Entries marked '*' are bibliographical entries rather than—or as well as—references.

*Austin, C.R. (1989) *Human Embryos*, Oxford University Press, Oxford.

Beauchamp, T.L. and Childress, J.F. (1989) *Principles of Biomedical Ethics*, 3rd edn, Oxford University Press, Oxford, p.315.

Birmingham Maternity Hospital (1989) *Annual Report.*

*Cox, Baroness (1991) Ethical issues for nurses. *Nursing*, **4**(34), 20.

Cuckle, H.S. and Wald, N.J. (1984) In *Antenatal and Neonatal Screening* (ed. N.J. Wald), Oxford University Press, Oxford, p.1.

*Dimond, B. (1990) *Legal Aspects of Nursing*, Prentice Hall, London, pp.88–89.

Fagot-Largeault, A. (1990) The notion of the potential human being, in *Philosophical Ethics in Reproductive Medicine* (ed. Bromham *et al*.), Manchester University Press, Manchester.

Gallagher, J. (1984) *The fetus and the law—Whose life is it anyway?* MIDIRS Information Pack No 3 (December 1986).

*Gillon, R. (1986) *Philosophical Medical Ethics*, John Wiley and Sons, Chichester, p.1.

*Green, J.M. (1990) *Calming or harming?* Occasional Papers, 2nd Series, No 2., Galton Institute, pp.32–33, 35.

*Harris, J. (1990) Wrongful birth, in *Philosophical Ethics in Reproductive Medicine* (ed. Bromham *et al.*), Manchester University Press, Manchester, pp.156–171.

HMSO (1967) *Abortion Act 1967*, Amended, HMSO, London.

*Kenny, M. (1986) *Abortion*, Quartet Books, London, pp.4–5.

King Edward's Hospital Fund for London (1987) *Screening for Fetal and Genetic Abnormality*, p.7.

Kuhse, H.and Singer, P. (1985) *Should the Baby Live?*, Oxford University Press, Oxford, p.10.

Lilford, R. and Thornton, J. (1990) What is informed consent?, in *Philosophical Ethics in Reproductive Medicine* (ed. Bromham *et al.*), Manchester University Press, Manchester, p.213.

Morgan, D. and Lee, R.G. (1991) *Blackstone's Guide to the Human Fertilisation and Embryology Act 1990*, glossary, Blackstone Press, London, pp.4–5.

Mosby (1986) *Mosby's Medical and Nursing Dictionary*, C.V. Mosby, St Louis, USA.

*Pratt, R. (1991) Moral decision making in the age of Aids. *Nursing*, **4**(34), 17.

*Richards, M.P.M. (1989) Social and ethical problems of fetal diagnosis and screening. *J. Reproduct. Infant Psychol.*, **7**, 171–185.

6.

MATERNAL VERSUS FETAL RIGHTS

CASE STUDY

Two weeks ago, following an antenatal clinic appointment at the hospital, Anola, a 28 year old expecting her second baby, was very anxious as she travelled home. On her arrival at the house she was greeted by her mother Pearl who was taking care of Anola's two-year-old daughter. The mother quickly assessed that her daughter was upset and, 'fearing the worst', she sent her granddaughter out to play in the garden.

Anola explained what had occurred at the hospital: the midwife had thought that the baby was a 'breech', she had asked for the consultant's opinion and he had ordered an ultrasound scan to confirm it. She felt that the consultant—on receipt of the scan report—had been very good. He made sure that she understood what he was talking about. She told him that she was one of three children, all born to her mother by vaginal breech delivery. She was not worried until he stated that she would need a caesarean section, because of the baby's presentation.

The doctor explained that the baby might have difficulty negotiating her pelvis during labour but Anola could not understand why this should happen as she had already been delivered 'naturally' of a baby weighing seven pounds. Without trying to frighten her, the consultant explained that there were other possible complications in breech deliveries and that his policy was to perform a caesarean section at 38 to 39 weeks of pregnancy.

When Anola enquired as to the possibility of having the baby 'turned', she was told that this technique was very dangerous and not, therefore, performed at that hospital. She was told, however, that the baby could still turn by him/herself but that as she had reached 35 weeks of pregnancy, it was highly unlikely.

Anola was asked to make a further appointment for two weeks time, making sure that she went to see her own GP or midwife during the week in between.

Pearl shared her daughter's concern but could only refer to her own situation, having had three breech babies who were all normal. She also said that the doctor was the expert and that they should at least listen to him. This view was reiterated by Anola's partner Leonard on his return from work, although he felt he would be content to accept Anola's decision.

The next day, Anola contacted her community midwife. She explained the situation and asked if the midwife could visit. The midwife arrived that evening, armed with a doll and a model pelvis and some colourful charts. He listened to the views of the couple and explained a breech delivery (with the visual aids). He also explained the reasons why turning the baby—externo-cephalic version—was considered dangerous and the possible reasons for the consultant's policy with regard to breech presentation. Having tried to be unbi-ased in his explanations, the midwife told Anola that it would be her decision to make. He made arrangements to visit twice more before the next hospital appointment, giving plenty of time for questions to be asked and answered.

Today is Anola's appointment at the hospital. Leonard will accompany her because she feels nervous about informing the doctor of her decision to refuse the caesarean section, unless an actual problem occurs in labour. She feels con-fident, however, that it is the right decision for her and her baby.

Issues that are not discussed here, but which readers may wish to pursue, are privacy, externocephalic version and mode of delivery of a breech.

QUESTIONS FOR CONSIDERATION BY THE READER

1. Does Anola have the right to refuse the caesarean section?

2. What rights, if any, does the fetus have in this situation?

3. Can the obstetrician take any action to enforce the operation?

4. Will the baby have any rights, in relation to Anola's decision, after birth?

It is important to remember that when considering a fetus we are concerned with the end of the 8th week of pregnancy (Morgan and Lee, 1991) until birth, expected at around the 40th week. Although most initial formation has occurred by the end of the embryonic period, much development and growth takes place in the next 32 weeks. This could be relevant when considering what rights should or should not be endowed on the fetus.

It is fully accepted by the author that this actual case is not one where the midwife has a direct dilemma. However, this sort of situation can arise quite frequently and, as in this case, the midwife is responsible for giving support to the client in a number of ways. The discussion points regarding rights are obvi-ously transferable to many other situations, some of which may well create dilemmas for midwives.

Question 1. Does Anola have the right to refuse the caesarean section?

This question deals with Anola's rights. If she is considered to be a rational person then she is also considered to be autonomous; her autonomy gives her the right to make informed decisions, for instance the giving or withholding of consent to operate. (For further explanation, see the case study on 'Autonomy and consent'.) In this situation the operation is a caesarean section, suggested by the obstetrician, in order to protect the fetus from possible damage during a vaginal breech delivery. Anola has sought professional clarification from the consultant and her midwife and has, therefore, exhibited rational behaviour in seeking information prior to making a decision. It is necessary to consider whether this specific situation changes Anola's rights, i.e. whether one's individual liberty depends upon not harming others'. For instance, consideration of whether she loses her autonomy because the fetus is considered 'at risk'. This could be taken a step further by considering whether or not she would be expected to undergo surgery for the sake of her child once it is born. She could not be forced to donate a kidney to her child—assuming tissue matching is achieved—although Eekelaar (1988) suggests that:

> ... morality may well expect the parent to help, unless the procedure were life-threatening to the parent.

This suggests that Anola might be expected to give up all her rights—except her right to life—if this might benefit the fetus. It could mean losing control of her own body. Apart from decisions regarding the method of delivery of the fetus, it could be expected that she perform—or refrain from performing—certain types of exercise or activity. She may be expected to give up her personal choice of food and drink if it were considered that this would create a better environment for the fetus. This has already occurred with eggs (salmonella risk), paté, soft cheeses (listeriosis risk) and now liver (excess vitamin A). Drug usage—including nicotine and alcohol—has come under the medicosocial microscope for even longer. Women have a legal right to continue to work during late pregnancy—they are no longer expected to resign or take maternity leave from the end of the 28th week of pregnancy, which was, until 1 October 1992, the time of legal viability of the fetus. (It is currently the end of the 24th week.) Many employers, however, will only permit women to continue past this time with a doctor's certificate of fitness to continue. This appears to give doctors the opportunity to deny the woman her right to work, in favour of the fetus.

Sometimes doctors and midwives put pressure on women to stop working so that they can rest and increase the chances of good fetal growth. Apart from curtailing the freedom of these women, it could reduce their chances of earning much-needed wages. Also, it could lose them their jobs, particularly before the end of the 26th week of pregnancy, the lower employment limit for entitlement to maternity leave. Another right that may be infringed is that of privacy. This applies to bodily privacy, particularly with the number of examinations many pregnant women are subjected to, and also to the amount and type of information that women are requested to divulge.

Some people may consider these rights to be comparatively trivial, where there could be possible adverse effects on the well-being of the fetus by the woman disregarding the advice given. Others, however, may consider these rights to be fundamental and therefore not to be infringed, regardless of the outcome to the fetus.

Many people (lay and professional) would criticize a woman for refusing treatment that could benefit—or prevent damage to—her unborn baby. Presumably this criticism would be based on the view that a woman should naturally protect her fetus and agree to anything that is to the fetus' benefit. In this case, the suggested procedure holds risks for the mother, although it is hoped that the present day techniques for caesarean section—by general or epidural anaesthesia—have greatly limited the dangers. Unlike a child requiring transplant surgery, this particular fetus is not in a definite life-threatening situation, therefore the mother's refusal is not committing the fetus to die. She has in fact opted to take a small risk, based on the facts as previously given, and will probably consent to surgery if the actual need arises. It should be stated that there would also have been a risk to the fetus as well as the mother by performing a caesarean section.

Question 2. What rights, if any, does the fetus have in this situation?

The dilemma here is created by the apparent conflict between maternal and fetal rights. Whose rights must be considered to be paramount? Who should be considered first—the woman or the fetus? Legally the dilemma does not exist as the fetus has very limited rights. The rights afforded refer to the subjects of inheritance, congenital disability and personal injury, and are contingent on being born alive (Freeman, 1988).

As the law stands at present, the fetus is not legally considered to be any doctor's 'patient'. To be a [human] patient the fetus would need to have the status of a person; this status is not accepted until complete expulsion from the mother has occurred. Even then, to be considered a registrable baby—and therefore a person—the birth (live or still) must occur after 24 weeks or it must be a live birth before expected viability. A fetus born dead before 24 weeks is just that: a dead fetus, not a dead baby who is required by law to be registered, and is usually named. This is the legal position. To the family it is often thought of as a baby, and therefore a person, from confirmation of the pregnancy. It seems unreal to think that a few hours before the fetus/baby is born—even during labour itself—a fetus has no rights. The moment of birth is therefore more than a physical and emotional occasion, it actually bestows legal rights.

Question 3. Can the obstetrician take any action to enforce the operation?

This question relates to the obstetrician's powers of action and whether there is anything he (or she) can do to enforce the caesarean section, an action that might be possible if he were in the USA. As the law stands, as Anola is conscious and rational, the doctor cannot take any action. He is able but unlikely to refuse to continue with her case, as, when he accepted her into his caseload at the beginning of her pregnancy, he was agreeing to abide by the duties of his office. His practice should include observance of his patient's autonomy, therefore he should accept her informed refusal to elective caesarean section. What he must do, to protect himself from any future litigation in this case (presumably his main reason for suggesting caesarean section in the first place) is talk to her again to ascertain that she understands what she is doing, then document her decision in the case notes. In view of a British case that occurred in 1992 (Dimond, 1993) there is the possibility that the court could rule in favour of caesarean section if the consultant applied for it. This would probably only occur if a complication arose but Anola has already stated that she would reconsider if a problem occurred. Regardless of the legal situation, it must be said that it takes someone with great emotional strength to hold out against the informal power that medical staff wield.

Question 4. Will the baby have any rights, in relation to Anola's decision, after birth?

This final question refers to the limited rights indicated previously, particularly with regard to congenital disability. Under *The Congenital Disabilities (Civil Liability) Act 1976*, subsection (2)(a)(HMSO, 1976), a child who is born with a disability resulting from events that ...

> ... *affected the mother during her pregnancy, or affected her or the child in the course of its birth, so that the child is born with disabilities which would not otherwise have been present* ...

... can take legal action against the person(s) responsible, up to the age of 21 years. The action would obviously be taken on the child's behalf up to the age of 18 years, but as an adult that person would have to take action personally. In the case of a fetus presenting by the breech, if the consultant obstetrician favours vaginal delivery and the baby sustains brain damage or other injury from the delivery, then the consultant could be held liable. Much would depend on the exact circumstances of the case because, although there is bound to be evidence of a body of opinion in favour of both methods of breech delivery (vaginal and caesarean section), the accepted criteria would undoubtedly differ slightly between practitioners. The other professionals who could also be held responsible, are the midwife or doctor performing the actual delivery. They can, however, only be held responsible for any act or omission considered to be negligent in their conduct of the case, not for the policy decisions of the consultant.

In this case, Anola has rejected the obstetrician's recommendation as she apparently considers that a planned caesarean section is an unnecessary intervention. Provided the obstetrician has taken all reasonable steps to ensure her understanding of the situation and has made suitable recordings in the case notes, he cannot be held responsible for the outcome, that is assuming he takes all reasonable precautions required in a vaginal breech delivery, including good technique if he is conducting the delivery. However, this does not mean that the woman herself can be held legally responsible if injury occurs. Under the terms of this Act, the mother can only be held responsible for injury occurring to the fetus when she is driving a motor vehicle.

FURTHER DISCUSSION

Many women feel obliged to create a good environment for their foetuses. To this end they will usually forego elements of their liberty and 'obey the rules' relating to diet, rest, hygiene, medication and addictive drugs (including nicotine and alcohol) but the fetus does not have the 'legal right' to this environment (Kenny, 1986). Although the law aims to generally prohibit the termination of 'normal' foetuses after 24 weeks' gestation—except where the mother's health is seriously at risk—it has not offered any legal assistance in maintaining a good environment for these foetuses. Society appears to rely on the mother's perceived obligation regarding this. It may therefore be necessary to determine what the basic requirement is and what may be considered to be supererogatory.

Some women, of course, for reasons of ignorance, lack of understanding or purely through personal choice, do not try to create this environment in all or any of these aspects. In some cases, women may be well aware of the possible hazards of smoking and drinking alcohol while pregnant but feel that indulging in either or both of these habits is all that helps them to relax at the end of the day. If they feel that continued stress could affect their foetuses, they are likely to opt for continuing their habits. The midwife, doctor, or even a relative, may end up in a difficult position, wanting to protect the fetus but only able to offer advice and education. In some cases the professionals are able to exert some informal power by the fact that some members of the public will believe that a 'medical suggestion' *must* be obeyed.

It is difficult to determine why the fetus has only relatively recently become so important that public debate has been entered into. Perhaps it is because of the advances in technology, with ultrasound scanning showing expectant parents their 'babies' prior to the moment of birth. Also, the advances in fertility treatment have created the need for discussion to provide clarity over specific issues. Another possibility is that—as adults are becoming more aware of their own moral and legal rights—perhaps they are beginning to broaden the scope of their questioning to include the status of the fetus.

The legal rights have been discussed but it could still be asked whether the fetus has *moral* rights and here responses would vary widely. According to Lockwood (1985), in discussing when life begins, being born and registered does not create a 'person' as it 'is not a biological concept at all'. It seems reasonable to suppose that most people would accept that the endurance of birth, followed by registration, is insufficient to create such a difference in status between a fetus of late gestation and a neonate. He further explains this:

A person … must have the capacity for reflective consciousness and self-consciousness. It must have, or at any rate have the ability to acquire, a concept of itself, as a being with a past and a future.

Anola obviously fulfils the above criteria and therefore has moral rights. One such right is that of liberty. According to Mill (1859) this allows her to do whatever she likes so long as she does not cause harm to others. Pregnancy, by definition, is not simply a 'self-regarding act', there is an 'other' involved (the fetus). It is necessary to determine the status that this 'other' may have and whether it is analogous to another live human being.

A neonate certainly cannot be considered in the first part of Lockwood's statement but it does have the potential 'ability to acquire' the concept. One still has to ask whether this differs from the potential of a fetus. It is difficult to determine what is so different about this living being, between two points in time so close together, which only places a legal onus on this woman to protect and care for her baby once (s)he is born. Harris (1985) considers the potentiality argument to be somewhat flawed. Among other criticisms, he states that to consider the fertilized ovum as having the potential to become a life, indicates that the component parts of it—i.e. the ovum and sperm—must each be considered to have the same potential and therefore the same protection. This could have far-reaching consequences. There is also no certainty that life will be achieved from each fertilized ovum as spontaneous abortion could occur.

It would appear that the major problem lies in deciding at what stage rights could be conferred on the fetus. Some people take the view that from the time of conception the fetus is a potential person and should be afforded the same rights as an independent being. This would naturally prevent legal termination of pregnancy; it would also prohibit the use of certain methods of contraception—those that prevent implantation rather than fertilization. In *The Warnock Report* (1984), Warnock (1985) and the *Human Fertilisation and Embryology Act 1990* (HMSO, 1990), 14 days following fertilization is taken as the most likely commencement of [potential] personhood, based on the development of the primitive streak but it was not suggested that full rights be bestowed at this time. Other people may consider that the time of viability is a suitable landmark—legally this would be 24 weeks. We know that it is possible for a fetus to survive before this time, which was the underlying reason for the change in the abortion laws, reducing the upper limit to 24 weeks in most cases.

Regardless of the legal status, if the fetus should be considered to have moral rights then perhaps one will be the right not to be harmed. Women could find themselves legally restricted to certain 'dos and don'ts' during pregnancy and labour. Areas that might be considered in pregnancy are diet, smoking, alcohol intake, travel, type of employment and attendance at 'Preparation for Parenthood' classes. In labour it could be place and time (which virtually happens now for many women), method of pain relief and so on. This would be a removal of the woman's rights and would be placing the worth of a fetus above that of an already independent living person.

In the case study, Anola does not appear to be considering the conflict of rights; she has merely considered the situation that faces her and has made her own informed decision.

It could be envisaged that many people, professional and non-professional, would applaud the suggestion of fetal rights with regard to harmful practices. This could, however, be the start of the 'slippery slope', where consideration of fetal rights rapidly results in the overruling of maternal rights. Most women, however committed to their unborn babies, would not wish to see a 'police state' for pregnancy, a situation that appears to be looming across the Atlantic and may be about to start in Britain, following a ruling in October 1992. In this case the decision was taken to enforce a caesarean section on a woman who had refused on religious grounds, in order to save both mother and baby. The baby died (Dimond, 1993).

In some states of the USA it would appear that women lose many of their most fundamental rights once they become pregnant. There have been well-reported cases of courts ordering certain women to undergo caesarean sections and blood transfusions. One of the most alarming occurred in Washington DC in 1987:

> *Angela, a primigravida, was twenty-five weeks pregnant and was admitted to hospital, seriously ill, with cancer; she was aware of her prognosis. She and her doctor agreed on a recommended course of treatment which was intended to prolong her life, at least until twenty-eight weeks, in order to give her baby a chance of survival. The hospital, however, against the wishes of all parties, obtained a court order for immediate caesarean section. The baby died two hours after delivery and Angela died two days later; her death certificate cited the caesarean section as a contributory factor.*
>
> (Shearer, 1989; Pollitt, 1990)

This case created outrage among individuals and organizations in the USA, resulting in a Court of Appeals ruling that :

> *... a dying pregnant woman has a constitutional right to refuse to have a forced caesarean section to save the life of her fetus.*
>
> (Anon., 1990)

However, there are at least three states where women have been ordered to undergo caesarean section for the health of their foetuses: Colorado, Illinois and Georgia (Gallagher, 1984). There are a variety of other legal interventions, in various states, on behalf of the fetus. Women have also been arrested following delivery, if urine testing of their babies has indicated that they were taking illegal drugs during pregnancy.

In 1981, in Kentucky, a man was convicted of the first-degree murder of a fetus following a vicious attack on his wife. After a legal wrangle throughout various courts, this was eventually changed to illegal abortion on the grounds that a fetus had never been considered a person. It is interesting to note that in several states the criminal death of a fetus does equate to murder (Gallagher, 1984).

With the UK's *Congenital Disabilities (Civil Liability) Act 1976* (HMSO, 1976), it appears somewhat illogical that the driving clause alone should be included, with regard to maternal responsibility. It would seem more acceptable to either exclude it altogether, or to include other categories of irresponsible behaviour that could cause congenital damage, such as drug abuse. In fact, although drug abuse does not feature in this Act, action can be taken against women who are drug abusers in pregnancy. This follows the decision in the House of Lords, in December 1986, to uphold the care order on the baby of a drug-addicted woman. This established the principle that pregnant women can be held liable for the care of their foetuses. This principle can embrace actions other than drug usage, including the topics mentioned earlier, in the discussion regarding fetal rights. This situation not only creates the increased possibility that mothers could be sued by their children for maltreatment but also that care orders could be issued where a mother is thought to have maltreated her baby *in utero*.

It would probably be fair to say that many people have conflicting intuitions with regard to this subject. On the one hand they believe in the woman's autonomy and right to choose—as in Anola's circumstances—and with abortion, but on the other hand they may feel that it is proper justice that certain crimes against the fetus be punished. They may also decry the woman who is a drug user for abusing her unborn child. Perhaps we need to determine a middle road in some way, one where the fetus can be afforded rights without a great deal of infringement on women's freedom. It seems fairly certain that if the British legal system continues to follow the precedent set in the USA, then women's rights will again become an explosive issue.

APPLYING THE THEORIES

A utilitarian view of maternal rights

A pregnant woman should have rights equal to any other person; she does not become less of a person because of her physical change of status. To infringe those rights, particularly for the sake of a fetus who legally has no rights, would be wrong. However, if the fetus were awarded certain rights—the observance of which would not infringe those of the mother—then extra 'good' would be created.

A deontological view of maternal rights

Although there is great debate surrounding the point at which life begins, deontologists believe that certain duties are owed to all 'persons'—such status not yet afforded the fetus. For this reason, it is unlikely that a deontologist would support the infringement of a woman's rights, despite the concerns relating to the sanctity of life. As with the utilitarian view, it would possibly be preferred if the fetus were awarded some rights without interference with those of the mother.

SUGGESTED READING

Carter, B. (1990) Fetal rights—A technologically created dilemma. *Professional Nurse*, **5**(11), 590–593.

Gallagher, J. (1984) *The Fetus and the Law—Whose Life is it Anyway?* MIDIRS Information Pack No 3 (December 1986).

HMSO (1967) *Abortion Act 1967*, amended, HMSO, London.

HMSO (1976) *The Congenital Disabilities (Civil Liability) Act 1976*, HMSO, London.

HMSO (1990) *Human Fertilisation and Embryology Act 1990*, HMSO, London.

Manning, M. (1987) How much guilt should a mother bear? *Nursery World*, 18 December 1986–1 January 1987, 8–10.

Pollitt, K. (1990) Tyranny of the foetus. *New Statesman*, 30 March, 28–30.

Shearer, B. (1989) Forced cesareans: The case of the disappearing mother. *Int. J. Childbirth Ed.*, **4**(1), 7–10.

REFERENCES

Entries marked '*' are bibliographical entries rather than—or as well as—references.

Anon. (1986) Rights in the womb. *The Times*, 5 December.

Anon. (1990) A major victory. *Birth*, **117**(3), 164.

*Areen, J. (1989) Limiting procreation, in *Medical Ethics* (ed. R.M. Veatch), Jones and Bartlett Publishers, Boston, USA, pp.94–123.

*Byrne, P. (ed.)(1990) *Medicine, Medical Ethics and the Value of Life*, John Wiley and Sons, Chichester.

*Carter, B. (1990) Fetal rights—A technologically created dilemma. *Professional Nurse*, **5**(11), 590–593.

*Chavkin, W. and Kandall, S.R. (1990) Between a 'rock' and a hard place: Perinatal drug abuse. *Pediatrics*, **85**(2), 223–225.

Dimond, B. (1993) Client autonomy and choice. *Modern Midwife*, **3**(1), 15–16.

Eekelaar, J. (1988) In *Health, Rights and Resources* (ed. P. Byrne), King's Fund Publishing Office.

Engelhardt, H.T. (1982) Medicine and the concept of person, cited in J. Areen, *Limiting Procreation*, as above, pp.94–123..

*Faulder, C. (1985) *Whose Body Is It?*, Virago Press, London.

*Freeman, M.D.A. (ed.)(1988) *Medicine, Ethics and the Law*, Stevens and Sons, London, p.10.

Gallagher, J. (1984) *The Fetus and the Law—Whose Life is it Anyway?* MIDIRS Information Pack No 3 (December 1986).

*Gaskin, I.M. (1987) More on court-ordered cesareans. *The Birth Gazette*, **3**(3), 20–21.

*Gillon, R. (1986) *Philosophical Medical Ethics*, John Wiley and Sons, Chichester.

Harris, J. (1985) *The Value of Life*, Routledge and Keegan Paul, London, pp.11–12.

HMSO (1929) *Infant Life (Preservation) Act 1929*, HMSO, London.

HMSO (1967) *Abortion Act 1967*, amended, HMSO, London.

HMSO (1976) *The Congenital Disabilities (Civil Liability) Act 1976*, HMSO, London.

HMSO (1990) *Human Fertilisation and Embryology Act 1990*, HMSO, London.

*Johnson, A.G. (1990) *Pathways in Medical Ethics*, Edward Arnold, London.

*Kenny, M. (1986) *Abortion*, Quartet Books, London, pp.4–5, 248–249.

*Lockwood, M. (ed.)(1985) *Moral Dilemmas in Modern Medicine*, Oxford University Press, Oxford, p.10.

*Mahoney, J. (1990) The Ethics of Sex Selection, in *Medicine, Medical Ethics and the Value of Life* (ed. P. Byrne), John Wiley and Sons, Chichester, pp.141–157.

Manning, M. (1987) How much guilt should a mother bear? *Nursery World*, 18 December 1986–1 January 1987, 8–10.

Mason, J.K. and McCall Smith, R.A. (1987) *Law and Medical Ethics*, Butterworths, London.

Mill, J.S. (1859) Introductory, in *On Liberty* (ed. S. Collini, 1989), Oxford University Press, Oxford.

Morgan, D. and Lee, R.G. (1991) *Blackstone's Guide to the Human Fertilisation and Embryology Act 1990*, Blackstone Press, London, pp.xi, 4–5.

*Pollitt, K. (1990) Tyranny of the foetus. *New Statesman*, 30 March, 28–30.

*Pratt, R. (1991) Moral decision-making in the age of Aids. *Nursing*, **4**(34), 17.

*Shaw, T. (1986) Limited rights for the unborn. *Daily Telegraph*, 13 October.

*Shearer, B. (1989) Forced cesareans: The case of the disappearing mother. *Int. J. Childbirth Ed.*, **4**(1), 7–10.

*Tooley, M. (1972) Abortion and infanticide. *Philos. Public Affairs*, **2**(1), pp.57–85.

Warnock, M. (1985) *A Question of Life*, Blackwell, Oxford.

7.

RESOURCE ALLOCATION

CASE STUDY

Longshot General Hospital serves an inner city population. The fairly large Maternity Unit provides the relevant care and facilities for 4000 deliveries per year. It also incorporates the gynaecological service.

Recently the hospital was offered a large sum of money from a benefactor on condition that it be used to set up an NHS 'assisted reproduction programme'. This was to include procedures such as gamete intrafallopian transfer* and *in-vitro* fertilization†.

The donation was sufficient to cover the initial outlay but the ongoing costs would have to be met by the existing obstetrics and gynaecology budget. Some members of staff were delighted at the prospect of NHS provision of reproductive technology, others were concerned at the lack of provision, already experienced, of sufficient, up-to-date equipment and facilities for the existing client case load.

After much deliberation, the health authority declined the offer. They were aware that the sum of money would have bought new equipment—some of which could also have been used in the existing service—but they could not justify the expense of the revenue consequences from an already stretched budget. While they sympathized with the infertile couples who might have benefited, they felt that their duty was to try to provide adequate facilities for the majority of clients rather than special services for the few.

QUESTIONS FOR CONSIDERATION BY THE READER

1. What effects might this programme have had on the existing service?

2. If some of the equipment could have been used for the existing clients, should this have been a major consideration?

3. What are the implications of income generation and should treatment depend on individual resources?

---

* Gamete intrafallopian transfer is the process by which the ova are retrieved from the ovaries abdominally, then replaced with the sperm into the fimbriated end of either or both fallopian tubes. Fertilization therefore occurs within the woman's body—if successful.

† *In-vitro* fertilization is the process by which the ova are retrieved, then placed, with the sperm, in a culture dish. Fertilization therefore occurs outside the woman's body—if successful. Resulting embryos are transferred to the uterus for implantation.

4. If the health authority wanted to promote 'the greatest good for the greatest number of people', is it fair to say that, by assisting more couples to achieve desired pregnancy, an even greater number of people could have been satisfied?

5. Do people have a right to have a child?

In order to consider questions 1 to 3, readers would need to imagine themselves in the position of the health authority members and to what they would have given consideration.

Again, it is accepted that this case does not pose a midwifery problem, but it is essential for midwives to understand something of the background thoughts regarding resource allocation, especially if they are to become effective managers. Infertility is a suitable topic to consider in this regard as it is becoming more common for midwives to see women who have undergone some means of fertility treatment.

Issues that are not discussed here, but which readers may wish to pursue, are selective abortion in multiple pregnancy, gamete donation, surrogacy, embryo research and eugenics.

Question 1. What effects might this programme have had on the existing service?

The case study states that the donation would cover the total outlay. In reality this is rarely the case but it can be assumed that it is true for this exercise. The financial problems would occur once the scheme was underway, by way of the revenue consequences occasioned by the scheme itself. Salaries and training costs would undoubtedly account for a major portion of these expenses, but some of the other areas to consider are the overheads on the accommodation, running and maintenance costs of technical equipment, and the cost of disposables and glassware. There would also be the 'hotel' costs created by any in-patient.

It is possible that the donation was sufficient to build new accommodation, but unless it was adjacent to the existing hospital, more services would be required. Use of existing premises—with appropriate alteration—would require less duplication of services, but consideration must be given to the available space and the ability of existing services to accept the additional work. The authority should have considered existing workloads and the effects that this increase would have. It is possible that the present funded establishment could cope with the expansion, at least initially, and therefore extra salary expenditure would be saved. However, there is every possibility that staffing is already stretched and unable to undertake an extra load, but even if they could, many of the staff already in a post would probably require additional training, which would deplete the existing levels. (Similar situations have occurred with Macmillan Nurses, where initial outlay has been covered but then the service has been left to cope within existing funds.)

The waiting lists could definitely get longer if the same theatre time and staff were used for all cases. It could be foreseen that the public may blame this expensive programme for any shortfall in local health services generally, and perhaps would not accept explanations regarding the finer points of hospital budgeting. Carver (1989) is one of many who have given voice to society's question of whether or not it is right that vast amounts of money:

> *... be expended on achieving pregnancies in infertile couples when there are many diseases and conditions affecting much larger sectors of the population that are underresearched and underfunded.*

Also adequate and appropriate counselling services are essential, and, because of the nature of the work, time-consuming. Not only is this service necessary when problems occur during pregnancy, labour or the postnatal period, but before treatment starts and certainly if it fails!

If we take 10% to be the figure for infertility (as it is the median of suggested figures; see 'Further discussion'), the health authority needs to consider the views of the remaining 90% of the local population. Some will undoubtedly be against the proposal of such facilities, feeling perhaps that it is 'going against nature', this view being held by some on religious grounds; others might feel instinctively that it is 'wrong'. Many would probably hold the view that it is up to the individuals themselves, that they have the right to bear children if they want them, and that public opinion should not be considered. What would their views be, however, if—following the initiation of the programme—the situation arose where all women having had normal deliveries of healthy babies were transferred home on day one or two after the birth because the obstetric ('obs') unit could no longer afford to offer a longer stay; or the waiting list for hysterectomies and other gynaecological ('gynae') surgery became longer? This could occur because the ongoing infertility costs would be met from the same budget as the two examples given.

Question 2. If some of the equipment could have been used for the existing clients, should this have been a major consideration?

This concerns the fact that some of the necessary equipment could have been used for existing clients. This may suggest good use of resources—covering a greater number of patients/clients—but determination of which 'existing clients', treated from the obs and gynae budget, would benefit from such equipment is necessary. The majority would be infertile couples already undergoing investigation and more conservative treatment, perhaps prior to referral to larger, more technical centres. The increased amount of equipment would only assist these couples if there was an adequate increase in the staff required to use it. Items such as laparoscopes and scanners might well be of use for other gynae patients undergoing abdominal investigation, with scanners also being used for fetal scanning.

If existing services were being used—as opposed to a new, purpose-built unit—then treating more gynae cases with the increased equipment would create greater competition for theatre and scanning time. This would probably result in less infertility treatment than the benefactor would have anticipated. If a new theatre were built and more staff were employed, there would still be problems as sharing equipment between two or more theatres—or scanning departments—is inadvisable. Realistically, it is more probable that the infertility services would require to use all equipment to the exclusion of other cases. This does not indicate the 'good value for society' previously mentioned.

Question 3. What are the implications of income generation and should treatment depend on individual resources?

Financial difficulties have been highlighted, but this question suggests that there is a possibility that the suggested programme could generate income that would offset some of the expenditure. The donation was to set up an NHS programme, not a private one. However, some NHS programmes require donations of minimum amounts of money. A minimal charge is unlikely to cover much when consideration is given to the cost of private treatment, which varies from centre to centre: The Cromwell Centre for IVF and Fertility charges £95 for initial consultations, followed by £1750 per *in-vitro* fertilization cycle, which is not inclusive of hormonal medication (Cromwell Hospital, 1992). These amounts must surely encompass the profit margins associated with private care and this needs to be considered if income generation is to be achieved. Some private clinics are subsidized by academic (or other) funding; this benefits clients financially. One such centre, based at Birmingham Maternity Hospital, is able to set its fees at £35 for consultations, followed by £1000 per *in-vitro* fertilization cycle with a 6 to 12 month wait, or £1200 for immediate treatment (University of Birmingham, 1993).

Once a sum of money is mentioned, whether it is called a fee or a donation, it could be considered akin to kidnapping. In this case, however, it is not: 'If you want to see your child again, leave £x!.. .', but: 'If you ever hope to *have* a child—pay up!'. The idea of expecting these couples to pay, even a donation, would be immoral to some people. Perhaps a donation of about £200 would not be considered too much for the average couple to pay for *in-vitro* fertilization— if it is successful—but:

> In Britain, overall success is estimated at between eight and 10% ...
> (Spallone, 1990)

For the majority, therefore, it is not simply one payment that would be requested. It could be said that the idea of income generation in such an emotive area is at least amoral, if not immoral, as some couples would be unable to make use of the service through lack of financial backing; others would become financially embarrassed, possibly leading to a breakdown in a previously sound relationship. Yet Mrs Jane Denton, Director of Nursing at the Hallam, where the above private fees are charged, believes that:

> *If you are committed,* in-vitro *fertilisation isn't beyond the reach of most people.*
>
> (Trevelyan, 1990)

Johnson (1989) highlights something which, for some, could be similar to this situation in moral terms, in a chapter entitled 'Ethical issues in organ transplantation':

> *The ability to save specific lives, in a highly visible way, by transplantation raised the question whether any individual should be allowed to die because he or she could not afford the high costs of transplantation.*

Presumably this situation could occur in the USA where Johnson works but, as we know, this type of treatment is covered by the NHS here. This poses another question: why is it that the technological infertility treatments are 'private' but organ transplants are NHS funded? The obvious answer is that people would die without the transplants but why should their expensive needs be met rather than those of the infertile? Denton (cited in Trevelyan, 1990), it would appear, believes it is a mark of commitment. The author would argue strongly in favour of the afflicted couples, that they already exhibit sufficient commitment to their search for parenthood. Without it they surely could not continue on what is—for most people—such an arduous programme. If the payment is not to exhibit commitment, then perhaps it is because the treatment is considered a luxury, something most people would agree that individuals should fund for themselves. Transplants are for physical health, therefore they are considered essential; an item that is non-essential would probably be considered a luxury. It seems unlikely that we should accept this view, after all they are only seeking what most couples can choose to have at far less expense. In fact, some couples have far more than they can adequately cope with!

Perhaps a system should be introduced whereby couples could have babies by whatever method is necessary (e.g. naturally, *in-vitro* fertilization, surrogacy) so long as they have the necessary financial backing. This, of course, would be allowing the privileged members of society to have families—as is the present case with *in-vitro* fertilization—while the less fortunate couples would be hard pressed to raise the finances (again, as it is now). With assisted reproduction we are not allowing someone to die if they cannot afford treatment, rather we are denying them the assistance to produce a new life. It surely cannot be right that those who are less well off should be denied the life chances that the better off can afford? Perhaps a means-tested system could be introduced; this would seem a fairer method to some but undoubtedly there would be those against it. It still would not compensate for the natural injustice that many couples feel they have suffered, nor would it prevent the feeling that babies were almost being bought, the actual practice of which has been illegal since 1926 (Richards, 1989). It is illegal for money to change hands in cases of adoption and, although couples undergoing treatment with their own gametes cannot be said to be in the same situation, it could be said that those cases where donor gametes are involved are verging on it.

There is another possibility: that of insurance companies providing 'infertility insurance' policies. If this occurred, couples attempting to get such cover, once there is even the suggestion of a possible problem, would probably face exorbitant premiums, just as it used to be with 'twins' policies.

Question 4. If the health authority wanted to promote 'the greatest good for the greatest number of people', is it fair to say that, by assisting more couples to achieve desired pregnancy, an even greater number of people could have been satisfied?

This suggests that this is the authority's chance to increase its efficiency in creating good or happiness, almost like 'thermometer readings' of donations to charity appeals. In that situation the amount just grows according to the income—in the NHS it is very different. It is rarely possible to create good or happiness in health matters without it costing money. The NHS purse is not bottomless, therefore anything with a price tag depletes the resources. It is not possible to meet all requests and therefore keep the 'mercury of happiness' rising—it is more usual to have to transfer from one area to another so that, as one area benefits, so another goes without. In this case study the purse has been temporarily filled to the top, therefore an initial increase in happiness by way of the new programme might be achieved, but not as an ongoing process. Economists are expected to consider cost-effectiveness and efficiency, but it would appear that those in health care also consider the importance of doing more good than harm. Others may also do this but it is irrelevant here. This is the principle of utility—those who follow this principle are utilitarians (see Part One). The decision that was made regarding the assisted reproduction programme was basically utilitarian, but the last question is still to be answered: Were they right to decline the offer?

In order to decide whether or not couples suffering infertility could be accommodated within the budget, it is necessary to apply the three stages of the QUALYS approach (see 'Further discussion'). As with other conditions, investigations would be carried out on both partners and the actual cause diagnosed where possible. The next step is to decide whether the fault can be corrected quickly.

Undoubtedly many will not be easily rectified. Here the comparison of projected outcomes occurs: whether without treatment either partner will become worse or die. Obviously this would not be the case, at least not directly. The chance of a successful outcome if treatment is given will also be considered. This will depend on the problem—some cases are treatable with minor surgery or drug therapy and improved knowledge of the menstrual cycle. In such cases NHS treatment is usually offered. There will be some, however, that are unknown quantities, treatment such as superovulation together with *in-vitro* fertilization or gamete intrafallopian transfer may be successful, but the envisaged time span is uncertain, as is the place where the treatment can be obtained. There are very few NHS locations for this level of assisted reproduction, therefore the couple could be refused treatment, even if their health authority were prepared to pay for the service, as would be required under the new contract system.

In assessing value—which is part of creating the 'greatest good'—treatment must be cost-effective by achieving its objective with least resources. It is highly unlikely that this achievement could be predicted. There is a possibility of achieving a pregnancy after one course of treatment but as ...

... only about 10% of healthy-looking embryos successfully implant...
(Winston, 1989)

... and as few as 1–2% in newer units ...
(Austin, 1989)

... this is unlikely. The cost is also high, therefore it would appear that value could not be proved to an economist.

Question 5. Do people have a right to have a child?

One may question the principle of considering the many as opposed to the few, or the individual, and whether the 'greatest good' is most important. If it is, then the importance of the rights of individuals should be considered. In this question you are asked to consider the rights of the infertile couple and whether they have the right to fulfil all bodily functions. If they do, then perhaps they have the right to expect NHS treatment, whatever that entails, just as they would for medical and surgical problems. This leads to the question of whether people have the right to have a child. If the answer is considered to be 'Yes' then surely this means *all* people—that would include single women and single men, despite the sexual persuasion of either sex. The author would suggest that many individuals would not be in favour of this practice—whether the person is homosexual or not—but to formulate conditions is suggesting that not everyone has that right, therefore we would be guilty of discrimination. It would, perhaps, be more correct to say that people who want children do not have a right to them, more a natural desire for them.

It could also be suggested that reproductive technology has been responsible for a 'created want' of children, almost in the way that advertising succeeds in creating 'wants' (Poff, 1989). Carver (1989) calls it:

... exalting the desirability of a 'child of one's own' no matter how tenuous the connection of that child to the 'parents'.

It is possible that some people consider that there is a right to have a child, particularly within a stable relationship. It would be interesting to discover, however, whether they consider it to be equal to the right to basic health care. The author believes that most people would not choose to spend limited resources on infertility treatment at the expense of immunization and screening programmes, or free prescriptions for children, the elderly and certain other disadvantaged groups in society.

There is also the question of whether it is right to interfere with 'nature' in this way. While the practice is accepted by many, it should be realized that the Roman Catholic Church is just one of the religions that condemn most fertility interventions. It is particularly against the methods that include fertilization outside the woman's body or the use of donor gametes. This rules out *in-vitro* fertilization and any donor situation such as artificial insemination by donor, despite their belief that it is the duty of married Roman Catholic couples to produce families, particularly as artificial insemination by donor is considered equivalent to adultery.

It has previously been stated that the NHS purse is not bottomless. In order to be free from claims of bias or discrimination it is reasonable that health authorities provide the basic requirements for all patients/clients in the first instance, followed by the more common 'extras'—this would be the objective view. Subjectively, the high-powered and expensive treatments feel like the basics when it concerns ourselves and our families.

At one time couples either came to terms with not 'being blessed' with children, or they could fulfil their need for children by adoption. Unfortunately, for those who would be interested, there are very few babies for adoption these days. This also creates the problem of very tight criteria being set for approval of would-be adopters, making it an unrealistic option for most couples. Another option could be to attempt to correct the mental morbidity, not by assisting with reproduction but by assisting them to come to terms with childlessness. There is a support group where help and guidance can be sought—the National Association for the Childless—and there are many couples who have adjusted their life plans accordingly.

FURTHER DISCUSSION

Practical constraints to setting up an in-vitro *fertilization programme*

It is important to consider what must be achieved in order to receive the money offered. If it has to be an NHS programme of 'assisted reproduction', what does this entail? Facilities would be required for investigation, diagnosis, counselling and treatment of infertility, in those requiring these services, across the full range of techniques. These facilities would include out-patient, in-patient and theatre accommodation, equipment and technical services (e.g. pathology, radiology, etc.) for the various aspects mentioned, adequate staffing levels according to the skill-mix requirements and any appropriate training. It would also be necessary to obtain a licence to be able to conduct the practice of *in-vitro* fertilization (HMSO, 1990).

Ethical considerations

The health authority is basically a caretaker and distributor of the health services in a defined area, constantly involved in the allocation of their share of the NHS financial 'cake'. A report prepared by a working party on the ethics of resource allocation in the health care system, states:

> *... ethical implications are to be found in all types of decision about resource allocation... . The decisions of a laundry-manager to purchase new blankets, of a clinician to initiate a new surgical treatment, of a Minister of State to introduce a new management structure for the health service —all express choices about relevant priorities. [...] None of these choices can be dismissed as entirely beyond ethical concern.*
>
> (Weale, 1988)

As a body, the health authority is answerable to the Regional Health Authority and the Government. This is partly because of the NHS structure of management, through which the health authority is upwardly accountable to the Regional Health Authority, and partly because the Health Authority Chairman is appointed by the Secretary of State to whom (s)he is also directly accountable. Some Government (DHS) directives are channelled directly to the health authority, failure to carry out these directives could result in the Chairman losing the post. It is also concerned, to some extent, about the views of the public being served—the Government calls this 'informal accountability downwards' (Day and Klein, 1987). This is partly achieved by the involvement of the Chairman of the Community Health Council, the local health 'watchdogs'. It is, perhaps, important to consider how much weight should be given to public opinion as opposed to expert opinion. The public tend to be swayed by emotive issues— very little captures the attention of householders more than a photograph in the local paper of a couple with their baby having waited perhaps 10 years and three attempts at *in-vitro* fertilization to achieve their success. However, very little enthusiasm is evident when it is suggested, for example, that an incontinence programme be set up, or information is given to highlight the plight of numerous men and women requiring hip or knee replacements. It is often the case that the most vocal section of society are those in their child-bearing years. It is therefore easier for them to imagine themselves suffering infertility than it is with the other problems mentioned—unless members of their own families have suffered in this way.

In this case would the local population agree that in the setting up of such a service—if a licence were granted—adequate prioritization had taken place? It would be fair to assume that the infertile couples who wanted to pursue the path of investigation and possible treatment would be greatly relieved but they are in the minority. The incidence of infertility in the UK is considered to be 5–10%, although Johnson and Everitt (1990) have suggested 10–15%.

These figures are determined by the uptake of fertility investigation and treatment. It is therefore uncertain how accurate they are as some couples may not seek assistance. (It could be argued that a percentage of those who choose, from the outset, not to have children may be infertile without any awareness of it, but this is irrelevant in this situation as surely it is the frustrated desire to have children that is in question.)

If the programme were initiated, then the relevant couples could seek assistance locally, possibly reducing travelling time and costs as well as the possibility of achieving a pregnancy. The possible success of the programme could create its own problems, however, as ongoing care will be required. There is a greater incidence of multiple pregnancy in 'treated' cases (Lovell, 1986; Vines, 1990; Manning, 1990) and, while these may solve some of the problems for these couples, there is the risk of increased perinatal mortality and morbidity. Added to the natural distress created by death, disease or abnormality, there is the problem that the maternity and neonatal units may not be equipped to cope. The possibility of multiple pregnancy in itself raises important ethical issues. Not only those who consider conception to be the beginning of life find this practice unacceptable—Robert Winston, an infertility specialist, does not hold this view of conception yet he is against high-order conceptions (Winston, 1989; Vines, 1990).

Pregnancies that are conceived naturally, as opposed to technologically, are most commonly the result of fertilization of the single ovum, produced during the ovulatory phase of the human menstrual cycle. In both *in-vitro* fertilization and gamete intrafallopian transfer, superovulation is stimulated by drug therapy, ova retrieval then takes place at the expected time of ovulation. In the case of *in-vitro* fertilization, fertilization takes place *in vitro* in the laboratory. At one time, where five or six ova were successfully fertilized, they were all returned to the woman's uterus. Doctors performing *in-vitro* fertilization are no longer at liberty to transfer more than three embryos or ova, however, as the Interim Licensing Authority has ruled against it.

Where gamete intrafallopian transfer is used, as previously explained, the ova and sperm are placed in the fallopian tube(s) where fertilization would normally occur—*in vivo*. Practitioners who use this method of treatment are not directed regarding the number of ova replaced. The *Human Fertilisation and Embryology Act 1990* ('the Act'; HMSO, 1990), while formalizing the licensing authority in respect of *in-vitro* fertilization and research, did not encompass gamete intrafallopian transfer. (The Act states, however, that 'guidance' may be given in the *Code of Practice* for licensees—the Act, 1990.)

Many professionals feel that this was an unfortunate omission, as there are reports of some specialists transferring four or more ova at one time (Vines, 1990). In fact, according to Manning (1990), one particular practitioner who was opposed to limiting the numbers, is reported to have recorded in a professional journal, his transfer of 'eleven or more'. She also states that in 1987, *in-vitro* fertilization and gamete intrafallopian transfer accounted for more than half the multiple births in the UK, each of the two methods resulting in two of the four sets of quadruplets, and that 228 *in-vitro* fertilization transfers in that year involved five or more ova. In order to prevent some of the disasters of high-order multiple pregnancy, some consultants advocate selective reduction. At the Eleventh Annual Paediatric, Obstetric and Psychiatric (POP) Conference, in London in October 1990, it was reported that a consultant at King's College uses a transabdominal injection of potassium chloride near the fetal heart to achieve the selected reduction.

It was also reported that an American study revealed that:

> ... where the reductions were from 2/4 to 1/2 (i.e. 191 fetuses reduced to 101 fetuses), there was a subsequent 5% fetal loss ...

and:

> ... where the reductions were from 5/8 to 2/4 (i.e. 111 fetuses reduced to 44 fetuses), there was a subsequent 50% fetal loss.

This practice opens up a debate of its own but it will not be dealt with further at this time.

The reason for transferring more than one or two embryos, or ova, was understandable. The doctors were concerned with giving that woman, or couple, the best possible chance of having a baby at the end of the process, one that is long and expensive (physically, emotionally, socially and financially). If, however, events have shown this to be unwise, then surely doctors should resist the practice. If such high-order multiple conceptions occur, then the pregnancy itself is at risk. The live births that follow successful multiple pregnancy are high-risk babies, often preterm with increased rates of morbidity and mortality. It could be argued that we have a duty to maintain those babies already conceived, and those delivered, rather than expend financial and manpower resources on expensive, possibly vain attempts to alleviate the problems of infertile people.

It could be said that where there is *in-vitro* fertilization there is research[‡] and to a certain extent that cannot be argued against. Even if a formal programme of experimentation and research is not in operation, records must be kept accurately and audits undertaken, therefore giving an ongoing picture

---

[‡] In this case the author means non-therapeutic research, where the findings will be of future benefit while being of no benefit to the embryo used for the experiment. *In-vitro* fertilization would not have started if not for this kind of research.

and creating the mechanism for retrospective studies. The issue of research/experimentation has been well debated, particularly recently, but it will not be dealt with further in this section.

As previously stated, public opinion should be considered but care should be taken to avoid acting purely emotively. It could be argued that if a service can be provided to help a section of society, however small, then the authority should agree to it. Unfortunately, the NHS functions within a limited budget and—according to Buchanan (1989)—most significant problems are surrounded by or include allocation of scarce resources. Scarce resources are explained as 'limited availability compared to demand' (Mugford and Drummond, 1989). If, as stated earlier, the health authority is a caretaker and distributor of these resources, then they are responsible for ensuring the best possible value from those resources. Mugford and Drummond also state:

> In a world where there are many competing uses for the same resources [there is a] need to demonstrate that allocating more resources to a (specific) field would represent good value for society, when compared with alternative uses...

It could be argued that the example in the case study lends itself to a utilitarian or consequentialist approach, favouring the view that the money required to fulfil the revenue consequences could be best used for the many, rather than the few. This decision may well have been reached with the aid of cost–utility analysis, the commonest method of which, at the present time, is *QUality-Adjusted Life-YearS* ('QUALYS') (Downie and Calman, 1987). This assessment mechanism was devised by Professor Alan Williams and considers costs incurred not only by service providers but also by patients and families. It has been suggested that this system is more scientific, as opposed to the more emotive approach previously used, and that this puts the medical profession in a better position to make decisions. The basic concept is that:

> ... adding to somebody's years of life is a health benefit.
> (Weale, 1988)

Treatments come in two 'packages'—they are either quick and intensive or slower and more extensive. The people who require either of these 'packages' can also be categorized:

- Those who receive treatment.
- Those who will be treated but must wait.
- Those who are denied treatment for some reason.

Decisions must be made regarding who fits into which category. Judgements can be approached methodologically with an emphasis on changes in degree of morbidity. In order to do this there is the need to identify, value and measure the possibilities.

In acute situations it is easier to identify the most suitable possibility than in chronic conditions. In a case of acute appendicitis it is usual for surgery to be carried out and, following a relatively short period of recuperation, the patient is back to a previous general health status—the cause of the good effect is the treatment. In many conditions, the benefits are less tangible with a more protracted timescale; this makes it more difficult to prove that the good effect was caused by the treatment, in part or at all. The question might be: would it have occurred anyway? Another means of identifying possibilities is to look at the projected outcomes, both with treatment and without. If a person's condition will improve—with or without treatment—then it would probably be seen to be a waste of resources to order any. If, however, the person will become worse, perhaps even die, then the decision to treat or not must be made. If the decision is made in favour of treatment then there is a price to pay—the cost of the necessary resources. In order to keep the costs to a minimum, more decisions have to be made regarding the most cost-effective method, place and time for this to be carried out.

When considering the value of the possibilities, a treatment is considered cost-effective if it achieves the objectives with least use of resources. If the budget is used properly, then effectiveness can be maximized and standards achieved in the least expensive way. Measurement is very difficult as health is hard to define. It is considered by many to be a state of physical, mental and social well-being; to others it is the absence of disease. These views should be reflected in the design of any measurement tool. It should also be recognized that there are many different interventions and care regimes, each of which may give diverse results.

Measurement of health status in infertility cases is controversial. Some would say that there is no physical illness to start with, therefore a decrease in morbidity would not be achieved. Alternatively, one or both partners is/are suffering a bodily dysfunction, therefore they could be considered to be suffering from disease in a broad sense. Caplan (1989) states:

Diseases do not always impair or threaten health. Some diseases are unpleasant and disabling but do not compromise the health of the individual who has them.

This should cover infertility, although it could also be argued that these individuals may actually develop stress and stress-related illness, therefore it is relevant to consider them in the QUALYS assessment, both physically—where appropriate—and mentally. According to Wales (1990), evaluation of quality of life is conducted by a combination of two factors: the degree of disability and the degree of distress. The disability factor appears to be associated with physical condition alone, therefore little account seems to be taken of the other aspects of health that could be affected in the case of infertility. Downie and Calman (1987) suggest that the aim of health care does not involve health promotion alone but 'promotion of wholeness'. For many couples this would include their ability to have children. It has been said that there are different interventions for many conditions—if this is one of those conditions, then there should be a determination of what other methods of treatment are available to create a feeling of wholeness.

Applying the theories

A utilitarian view

As previously stated, a utilitarian or consequentialist approach would favour the view that the money required to fulfil the revenue consequences could be best used for the many rather than the few.

A deontological view

Deontologists may well consider that each person has the right to reproduce, therefore deciding in favour of the infertility programme. However, there are a number of religions where the followers are against certain types of treatment that 'interfere with nature' a little too much—this could influence the final decision.

Suggested reading regarding resource allocation

Buchanan, A. (1989) Health care delivery and resource allocation, in *Medical Ethics* (ed. R.M. Veatch), Jones and Bartlett Publishers, Boston, USA.

Mugford, M. and Drummond, M.F. (1989) The role of economics in the evaluation of care, in *Effective Care in Pregnancy and Childbirth* (ed. I. Chalmers *et al.*), Oxford University Press, Oxford.

Weale, A. (ed.)(1988) *Cost and Choice in Health Care*, King's Fund Publishing Office, London.

Suggested reading regarding assisted reproduction

HMSO (1990) *Human Fertilisation and Embryology Act 1990*, HMSO, London.

References

The literature used in writing this chapter is worth reading. However, with regular advances being made in fertility treatments, it is important to read the most up-to-date books and articles.

Entries marked '*' are bibliographical entries rather than—or as well as—references

Austin, C.R. (1989) *Human Embryos*, Oxford University Press, Oxford, p.81.

*Beauchamp, T.L.and Childress, J.F. (1989) *Principles of Biomedical Ethics*, 3rd edn, Oxford University Press, Oxford, Chapters 1, 2 and 6, p.35.

Buchanan, A. (1989) Health care delivery and resource allocation, in *Medical Ethics* (ed. R.M. Veatch), Jones and Bartlett Publishers, Boston, USA, p.293.

Caplan, A.L. (1989) The concepts of health and disease, in *Medical Ethics* (ed. R.M. Veatch), Jones and Bartlett Publishers, Boston, USA, p.55.

Carver, C. (1989) The new—and debatable—reproductive technologies, in *The Future of Human Reproduction* (ed. C. Overall), The Women's Press, Toronto, Canada, p.56.

Cromwell Hospital (1992) *Schedule of Charges*, February.

Day, P. and Klein, R. (1987) *Accountabilities*, Tavistock Press, London, p.81.

*Downie, R.S. (1988) *Baby Making—The technology and ethics*, The Bodley Head, London.

Downie, R.S. and Calman, K.C. (1987) *Healthy Respect—Ethics in health care*, Faber and Faber, London, pp.86, 218–219.

*Gillon, R. (1986) *Philosophical Medical Ethics*, John Wiley & Sons, Chichester, Chapters 3, 4 and 5.

*Glover, J. (1988) *Causing Death and Saving Lives*, Penguin, London, Chapter 4, p.63.

HMSO (1990) *Human Fertilisation and Embryology Act 1990*, HMSO, London, p.201.

Johnson, A. (1989) Ethical issues in organ transplantation, in *Medical Ethics* (ed. R.M. Veatch), Jones and Bartlett Publishers, Boston, USA, p.246.

Johnson, M. and Everitt, B. (1990) *Essential Reproduction*, 3rd edn, Blackwell Scientific Publications, Oxford, p.350.

Lovell, B. (1986) A way of hope. *Nursing Times*, **82**(44), 26–29.

Manning, M. (1990) The painful gamete intra-fallopian transfer of life? *New Statesman and Society*, 11 May, 12–15.

Mugford, M. and Drummond, M.F. (1989) The role of economics in the evaluation of care, in *Effective Care in Pregnancy and Childbirth* (ed. I. Chalmers *et al.*), Oxford University Press, Oxford, p.86.

*Norman, R. (1983) *The Moral Philosophers—An introduction to ethics*, Oxford University Press, Oxford.

Poff, D.C. (1989) Reproductive Technology and Social Policy in Canada, in *The Future of Human Reproduction* (ed. C. Overall), The Women's Press, Toronto, Canada, p.219.

Richards, M. (1989) *Adoption*, Jordan and Sons, Bristol, p.75.

*Singer, P. (1989) *Practical Ethics*, Cambridge University Press, Cambridge.

*Smart, J.J.C. and Williams, B. (1988) *Utilitarianism For and Against*, Cambridge University Press, Cambridge.

Spallone, P. (1990) The cost of conception. *Nursing Times*, **86**(18), 28.

Trevelyan, J. (1990) The birth of a specialism. *Nursing Times*, **86**(18), 33.

University of Birmingham (1993) Price list, January.

Vines, G. (1990) Doctors warn of loophole in embryo bill. *New Scientist*, 31 March, 21.

Wales, J. (1990) Accounting for the quality of human life. *The Guardian*, 30 October, 6–7.

Weale, A. (ed.)(1988) *Cost and Choice in Health Care*, King's Fund Publishing Office, London, pp.17, 56.

Winston, R. (1989) *Getting Pregnant*, Anaya Publishers, London, pp.230, 237.

CONCLUSION

This book has been written with the underlying intention that it should be of practical use to student midwives, and the midwives and tutors involved in their education and training. The format is intended to be flexible enough to suit the wishes of each individual—for this reason it has not been constructed according to a particular model or within a specific curriculum outline. The case studies and examples contained in Chapters 2 to 7 have been formulated in order to apply certain ethical principles specifically to midwifery or a midwifery setting, in the hope that they will interest midwives at all levels.

The case studies have been piloted with student groups of various levels and—because of the results achieved—they have been incorporated into the midwifery education programmes within the college where the author is employed. One cautionary note, however, would be that, as with any topic, one should not assume a set level of background knowledge. The author fell into this trap herself when dealing with embryo research with a set of senior students. She had assumed wrongly that they would understand what was meant by 'the primitive streak', especially in view of the publicity surrounding the *Human Fertilisation and Embryology Bill* in 1990. This resulted in more time being spent on background embryology than had been intended.

Additional information, relevant theory and discussion points have been included. These should help student midwives to become more aware of the moral—and in some cases legal—rights of the women they care for. It is also intended to equip them for the decisions that they make in everyday life, while assisting in their ability to function autonomously within the official boundaries. Midwives need to be able to recognize moral conflicts and dilemmas; they also need to be able to draw on the relevant principles with which to solve them. However, if they are unsure about which major theory they wish to follow, my general advice would be in keeping with that of Walt Disney's character, Jiminy Cricket:

Always let your conscience be your guide.

(Washington and Harline, 1940, Bourne Inc.)

GLOSSARY

act-utilitarianism: the traditional form of utilitarianism where every single action is judged by its consequences.

autonomy: the capacity to be rational and in control of liberty and freedom.

battery: any physical contact without prior consent.

beneficence: to do good or to help, as in a doctor's duty to his patients.

casuistry: disentanglement and reordering of 'rules' in conflict.

categorical imperative: this is Kant's guidance on objective moral action where it is decided what one ought to want and one should be happy with it.

conflict, moral: a trial of strength between principles.

deontology: an ethical theory based on duty.

descriptivism: the view that moral judgements have descriptive meaning only.

dilemma: the problem created by the conflict of principles, where all the choices offered seem to lack total satisfaction.

emotivism: a theory concerned with the meaning of ethical terms.

ethics: the underlying reasons—or set of standards—that regulate behaviour.

implied consent: the assumption that certain positive actions indicate acceptance by the recipient.

informed consent: the uncoerced permission given by an individual—following consideration of sufficient information—for another to take action.

liberty: having the right to do as you please.

licensing authority: the Human Embryology and Fertilisation Authority (HEFA) responsible for the issuing of licenses for treatment, storage and research in connection with activities covered by the Act.

monism: a theory based on one supreme principle or duty.

moral: relating to the rights and wrongs of everyday living.

non-maleficence: to do no harm.

particularism: a belief in the development of moral sensibilities rather than reliance on formal theories.

paternalism: making decisions on behalf of those who are rational enough to make their own decisions.

pluralism: a theory based on more than one principle, with none being supreme.

prima-facie duties: specific duties of equal importance.

QUALYS (QUality Assisted Life YearS): a system of objective decision-making in health care.

rational: self-determining, self-controlled.

rule utilitarianism: a modification of act-utilitarianism, it assesses an act according to moral rules.

sanctity of life: the belief that life is sacred.

subjectivist: someone who believes moral attitudes are a matter of taste.

teleological: a doctrine that considers everything to have been created by God to serve mankind.

universalizability: a principle that tests the morality of a judgement by universalizing it.

utililitarianism: a theory based on the consequences of actions.

AUTHOR INDEX

SUBJECT INDEX